NUTRIB_ _ _ _ _
RECIPES FOR
HEART HEALTH

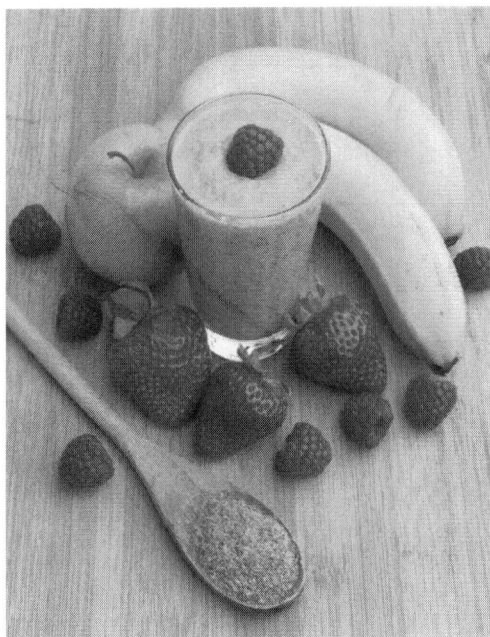

By

Celeste Jarabese

Celeste Jarabese

Copyright © CONTENT ARCADE PUBLISHING. All rights reserved.

This recipe book is copyright protected and meant for personal use only.

No part of this recipe book may be used, paraphrased, reproduced, scanned, distributed or sold in any printed or electronic form without permission of the author and the publishing company. Copying pages or any part of this recipe book for any purpose other than own personal use is prohibited and would also mean violation of copyright law.

DISCLAIMER

Content Arcade Publishing and its authors are joined together in their efforts in creating these pages and their publications. Content Arcade Publishing and its authors make no assurance of any kind, stated or implied, with respect to the information provided.

LIMITS OF LIABILITY

Content Arcade Publishing and its authors shall not be held legally responsible in the event of incidental or consequential damages in line with, or arising out of, the supplying of the information presented here.

Table of Contents

INTRODUCTION

This book is a part of a series of NUTRiBULLET recipe book that promotes Healthy Heart.

As we age, our body organs tend to weaken, especially if we don't lead a healthy lifestyle. Our heart for one, is a vital organ in the body that should be taken care of.

At present, cardiovascular disease is one of the major health concerns globally that has a high mortality rate. Sedentary lifestyle and faulty diets are the main reasons why people develop cardiovascular issues such as high cholesterol levels in the blood, atherosclerosis or also known as the hardening of the arteries, heart failure, and high blood pressure that can lead to stroke.To prevent these from happening, we should maintain healthy body weight, exercise regularly, and have a well-balanced diet that is also rich in fiber, vitamins, minerals, and antioxidants. Oneway to achieve that is by drinking healthy beverages like smoothies that contain these essential nutrients.

This book is for people who wants to maintain a healthy cardiovascular system and focuses on heart-friendly recipes. It includes a wide selection of smoothie recipes that calls for natural ingredients such as fresh fruits, vegetables, nuts, seeds, dairy, milk, and tea.

To help you further meat your health goals, the recipes in this book make use of an amazing machine called the

"NUTRiBULLETSuperfood Extractor". If you don't have it yet, now is the best time to buy one. This powerful machine will help you maximize the health benefits that you can get from your smoothies.

Let's get it on! Continue reading and I hope you get to try all the healthy recipes in this book.

Soy Yogurt Beet and Orange Smoothie

This delightful smoothie recipe with soy yogurt, beet, and orange can be taken at breakfast or snack. It will surely make your heart healthy and strong.

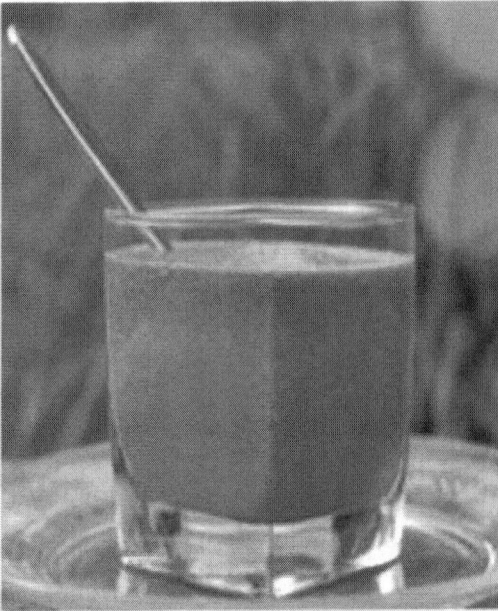

Preparation Time: 5 minutes
Total Time: 5 minutes
Yield: 1 serving

Ingredients

½ cup soy yogurt
1 medium beet root, diced
1 small orange, cut into segments
2 ice cubes
water to max line

Method

1.   Combine soy yogurt, beet root, orange, ice cubes, and water in the tall glass. Process in the NutriBullet for 20-30 seconds or until it becomes smooth.
2.   Pour in a serving glass. Garnish with a slice of orange, if desired.
3.   Serve and enjoy!

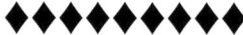

◆◆◆◆◆◆◆◆◆

Ginger Beet Fennel and Walnut Smoothie

This smoothie recipe with ginger, beet, fennel, yogurt, and walnuts is a great combination of flavor and good for you nutrients!

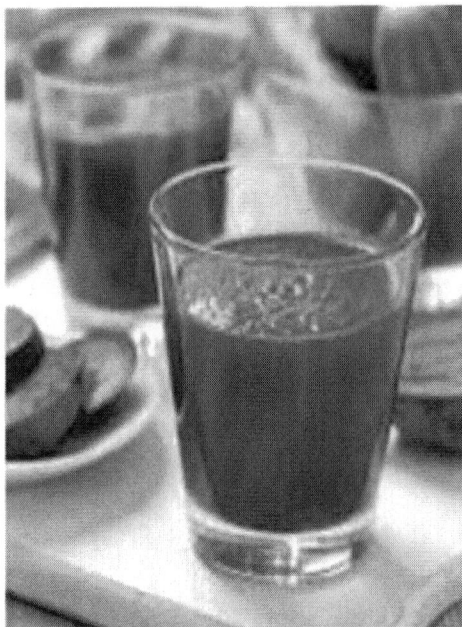

Preparation Time: 5 minutes
Total Time: 5 minutes
Yield:1 serving

Ingredients

1 medium beet root, diced
¼ medium fennel bulb, shredded
½ cup low-fat yogurt
½ teaspoon fresh ginger root, grated
6 pcs.walnuts
water to max line

Method

1.	Combine beet root, fennel, cucumber, low-fat yogurt, walnuts, and water in the tall glass. Process in the NutriBullet for 20 seconds or until it becomes smooth.
2.	Pour in a serving glass. Garnish with a slice of beet or sprinkle with grated ginger, if desired.
3.	Serve and enjoy!

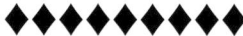

♦♦♦♦♦♦♦♦♦

Coconut Banana and Blueberry Smoothie

This tasty smoothie recipe with coconut milk, banana, and blueberries will provide your body with good amounts of healthy fats, carbs, vitamins and minerals which will keep you going for a long time.

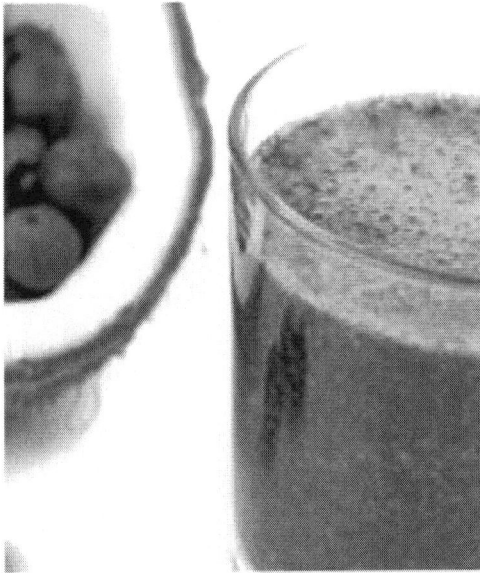

Preparation Time: 5 minutes
Total Time: 5 minutes
Yield: 1 serving
Ingredients

1 medium banana, cut into small pieces
½ cup blueberries
2 Tbsp. coconut milk
coconut water to max line

Method

1.   Combine the banana, blueberries, coconut milk, and coconut water in the tall glass. Process in the NutriBullet for 10-15 seconds or until smooth.
2.   Transfer mixture in a serving glass. Garnish with some blueberries, if desired.
3.   Serve and enjoy!

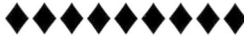

◆◆◆◆◆◆◆◆◆

Ginger Spiced Avocado Smoothie with Honey

This ginger-spiced smoothie recipe with avocado and honey is a nutrition packed beverage that you will definitely love because of its rich flavor and nutrition.

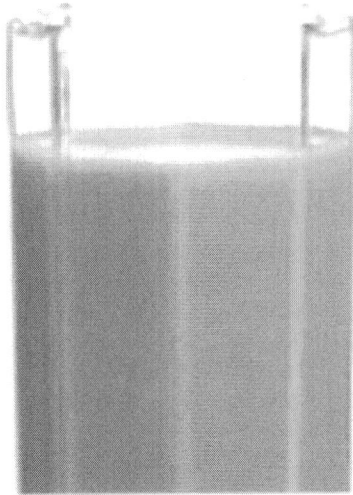

Preparation Time: 5 minutes
Total Time: 5 minutes
Yield:1 serving

Ingredients

¼ cup avocado, diced
2/3 cup skim milk
½ teaspoon fresh ginger, grated
1 teaspoon honey
water to max line

Method

1.   Place the avocado, skim milk, ginger, honey, and water in the tall glass. Process in the NutriBullet for 10-15 seconds or until smooth and creamy.
2.   Pour mixture in a serving glass. Sprinkle with some grated ginger on top, if desired.
3.   Serve and enjoy!

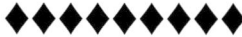

♦♦♦♦♦♦♦♦

Silken Tofu with Avocado and Kiwi Smoothie

This great tasting smoothie recipe with tofu, avocado, kiwi, and soy milk is the ideal recipe for you if you need a quick and healthy treat any time of the day.

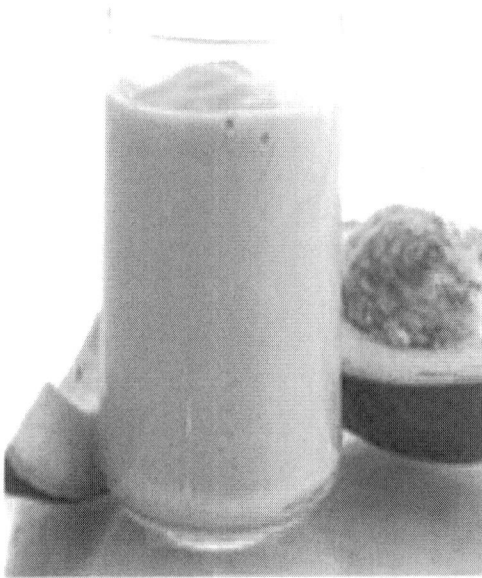

Preparation Time: 5 minutes
Total Time: 5 minutes
Yield: 1 serving

Ingredients

¼ cup silken tofu, soft
¼ cup avocado, diced
1 medium kiwi fruit
½ cup soy milk
1-2 ice cubes

Method

1.	Place the tofu, avocado, kiwi, soy milk, and ice in the tall glass. Process in the NutriBullet for 20-30 seconds or until it becomes smooth and creamy.
2.	Pour in a chilled tall glass. Garnish with a slice of avocado or kiwi, if desired.
3.	Serve and enjoy!

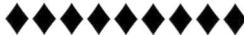

◆◆◆◆◆◆◆◆◆

Raspberry Pineapple and Kale Smoothie

This awesome smoothie with raspberries, pineapple, kale and almond milk can definitely give you the boost you need to fight sickness and keep your heart healthy.

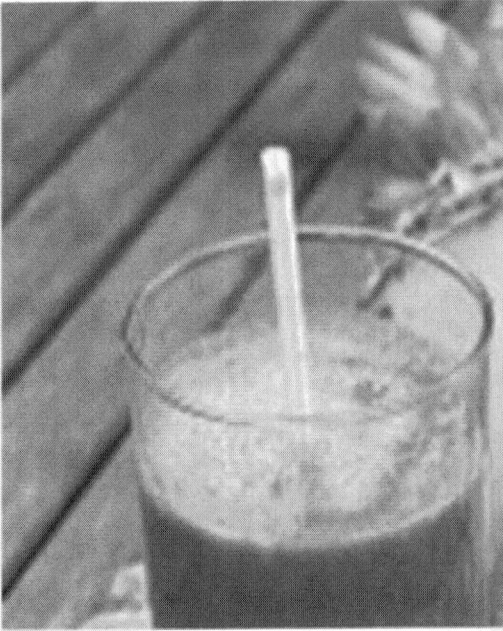

Preparation Time: 5 minutes
Total Time: 5 minutes
Yield: 1 serving

Ingredients

½ cup raspberries
½ cup pineapple chunks
1 handful kale, torn
2/3 cup almond milk

Method

1.   Place raspberries, pineapple, kale, and almond milk in the tall glass. Puree in the NutriBullet for 10-15 seconds or until becomes smooth and creamy.
2.   Pour in a chilled serving glass. Garnish with raspberries or pineapple, if desired.
3.   Serve and enjoy!

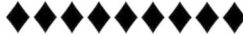

◆◆◆◆◆◆◆◆

Spiced Blackberry Soy and Oatmeal Smoothie

This smoothie recipe with blackberry, soy milk, oatmeal, and cinnamon is like a breakfast in a glass because it contains all the nutrients you need to start your day.

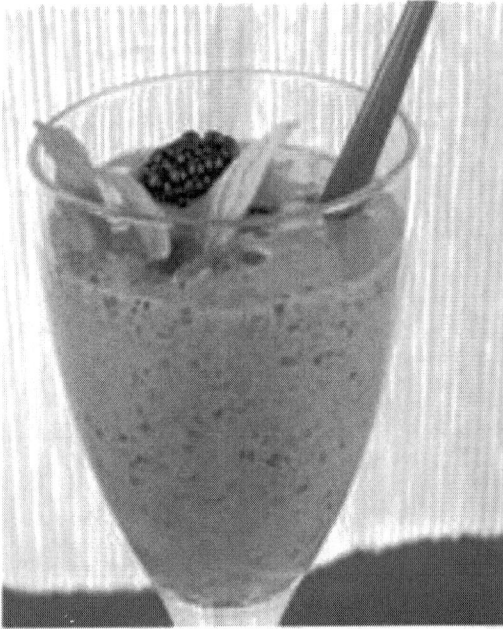

Preparation Time: 5 minutes
Total Time: 5 minutes
Yield: 1 serving

Ingredients
¾ cup blackberries
½ cup soy milk
¼ cup oatmeal, cooked, plain
¼ teaspoon cinnamon, ground
water to max line

Method
1.   Place blackberries, soy milk, oatmeal, cinnamon, and water in the tall glass. Process in the NutriBullet for 10-15 seconds or until combined well.
2.   Pour in a serving glass. Garnish with a few blackberries, if desired.
3.   Serve and enjoy!

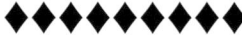

◆◆◆◆◆◆◆◆◆

Fennel Grapefruit and Hemp Seed Smoothie

A great tasting pink smoothie recipe that is full of nutrients that your body needs. You can make one in a snap and that it only requires some ingredients.

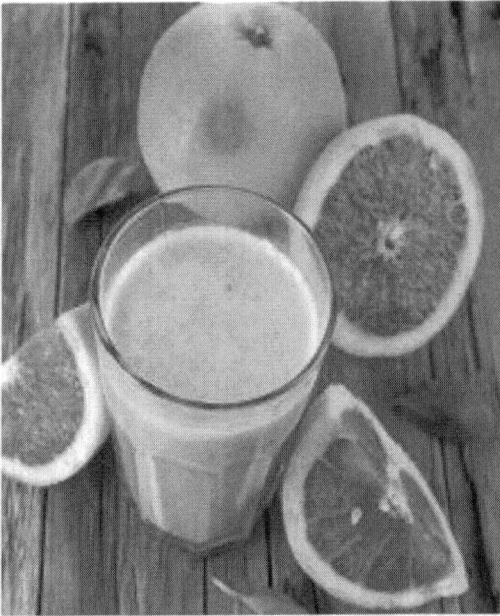

Preparation Time: 5 minutes
Total Time: 5 minutes
Yield: 1 serving

Ingredients

¼ medium fennel bulb, shredded
½ medium pink grapefruit, cut into
segments
¾ cup almond milk
1 teaspoon honey
1 teaspoon hemp seeds

Method

1.	Combine the fennel, grapefruit, almond milk, honey, and hemp seeds in the tall glass. Process in the NutriBullet for 10-15 seconds or until smooth.
2.	Pour in a chilled glass. Garnish with a slice of grapefruit, if desired.
3.	Serve and enjoy!

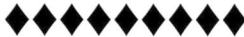

◆◆◆◆◆◆◆◆◆

Avocado Watercress and Lime Smoothie with Honey

This wonderful smoothie recipe made with avocado, watercress, lime, low-fat milk and honey will give you loads of nutrients to keep up with your active lifestyle.

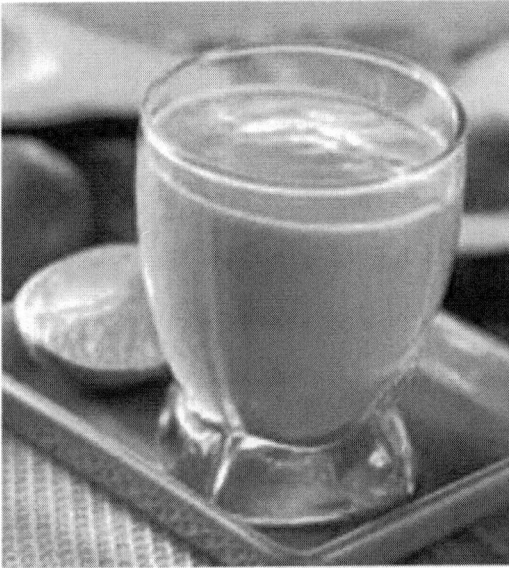

Preparation Time: 5 minutes
Total Time: 5 minutes
Yield: 1 serving

Ingredients

1/8 medium avocado, diced
1 handful watercress, torn
1 tablespoon lime juice
1 teaspoon honey
1 cup low-fat milk

Method

1.   Place the avocado, watercress, lime juice, honey, and low-fat milk in the tall glass. Process in the NutriBullet for 10-15 seconds or until it becomes smooth.
2.   Pour in a serving glass. Garnish with a slice of lime, if desired.
3.   Serve and enjoy!

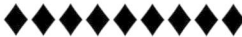

◆◆◆◆◆◆◆◆◆

Vanilla Blueberry Oat Smoothie with Chia

Looking for a great tasting breakfast on the go recipe? Well then, we've got you covered! This fiber-packed smoothie recipe is loaded with healthy goodness that can replace a complete breakfast.

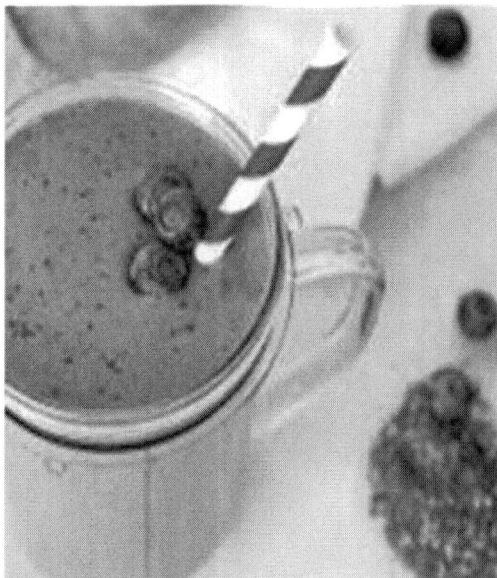

Preparation Time: 5 minutes
Total Time: 5 minutes
Yield:1 serving

Ingredients

½ cup blueberries
½ cup oatmeal, cooked
½ cup Greek yogurt
1 teaspoon chia seeds
water to max line

Method

1.   Place the blueberries, oatmeal, yogurt, chia seeds, and water in the tall glass. Process in the NutriBullet for 10-12 seconds or until it becomes smooth.
2.   Pour in a serving glass. Garnish with a few blueberries, if desired.
3.   Serve and enjoy!

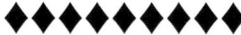

♦♦♦♦♦♦♦♦♦

Mango Kale and Pistachio Cooler

Need a heart-friendly drink? Well then you have come to the right place because this is the recipe for you! It is made with mango, kale, milk, and pistachio nuts.

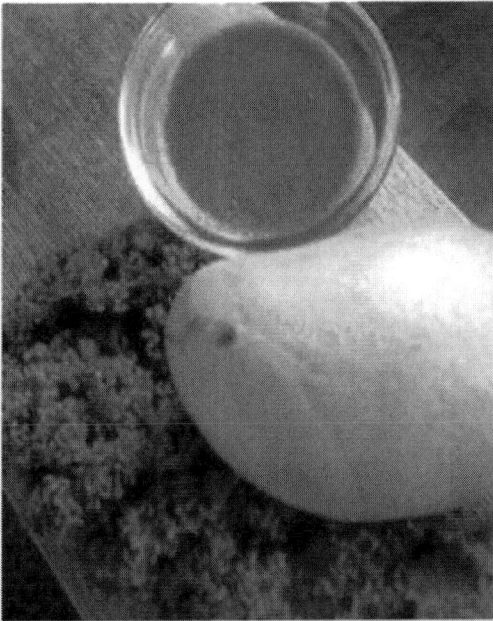

Preparation Time: 5 minutes
Total Time: 5 minutes
Yield:1 serving

Ingredients

¾ cup mango, diced
1 cup kale, torn
¾ cup skim milk
10 pistachio nuts
2 ice cubes

Method

1.   Place the mango, kale, skim milk, pistachios, and ice cubes in the tall glass. Process in the NutriBullet for 20-30 seconds or until it becomes smooth.
2.   Pour in a serving glass. Garnish with mango slices, if desired.
3.   Serve and enjoy!

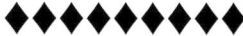

◆◆◆◆◆◆◆◆◆

Raspberry Walnut and Spinach Smoothie

This awesome smoothie recipe with raspberries, walnuts, and spinach is a must have especially when you are not feeling good. It will furnish your body with important nutrients to help you recuperate from sickness.

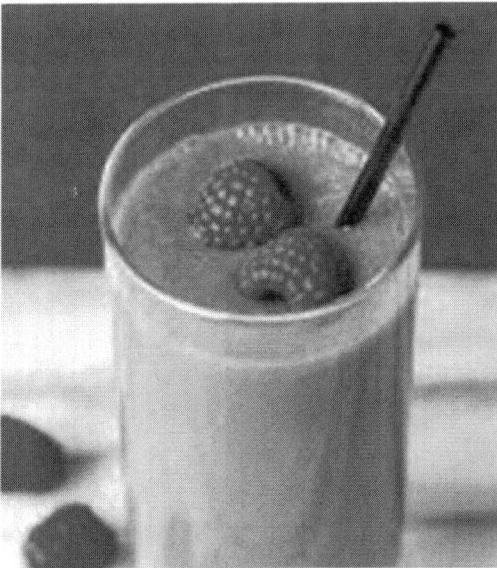

Preparation Time: 5 minutes
Total Time: 5 minutes
Yield: 1 serving

Ingredients
½ cup frozen raspberries
1 cup baby spinach
½ cup skim milk
1 teaspoon honey
6 walnuts
water to max line

Method
1.   Place the raspberries, spinach, milk, honey, walnuts, and water in the tall glass. Process in the NutriBullet for 10-15 seconds or until it becomes smooth.
2.   Pour in a serving glass. Garnish with a few raspberries, if desired.
3.   Serve and enjoy!

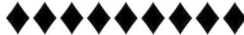

◆◆◆◆◆◆◆◆◆

Choco Almond Banana Smoothie

Craving for a chocolate shake? Try this healthy alternative to the usual calorie-laden smoothies. This recipe uses almond milk, banana, and cocoa powder.

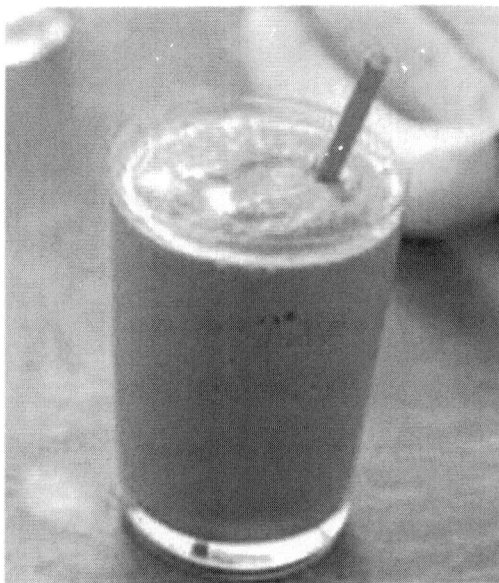

Preparation Time: 5 minutes
Total Time: 5 minutes
Yield: 1 serving

Ingredients

1 cup almond milk
1 medium banana, cut into small pieces
1 tablespoon cocoa powder
2 ice cubes

Method

1.   Place the almond milk, banana, cocoa powder, and ice cubes in the tall glass. Process in the NutriBullet for 20-30 seconds or until it becomes smooth.
2.   Pour mixture into a chilled glass. Garnish with banana slices, if desired.
3.   Serve and enjoy!

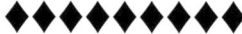

◆◆◆◆◆◆◆◆◆

Peach Banana and Tofu Smoothie

This nutrient packed smoothie recipe with peach, banana, and tofu makes a great on the go pre or post workout snack.

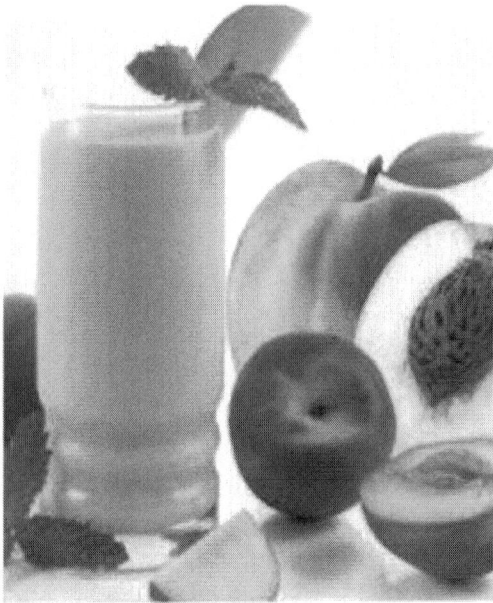

Preparation Time: 5 minutes
Total Time: 5 minutes
Yield:1 serving

Ingredients

½ cup peaches, peeled and diced
½ medium banana, cut into small pieces
¼ cup silken tofu, soft
½ cup soy milk

Method

1.   Place the peach, banana, tofu, and soy milk in the tall glass. Process in the NutriBullet for 10-15 seconds or until it becomes smooth and creamy.
2.   Pour in a chilled tall glass. Garnish with a slice of peach, if desired.
3.   Serve and enjoy!

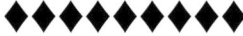

◆◆◆◆◆◆◆◆◆

Hawaiian Tropics Smoothie with Flaxseeds

This healthy and delicious smoothie with tropical flavors is made with papaya, banana, pineapple, and coconut. It is loaded with nutrients that are good for your heart.

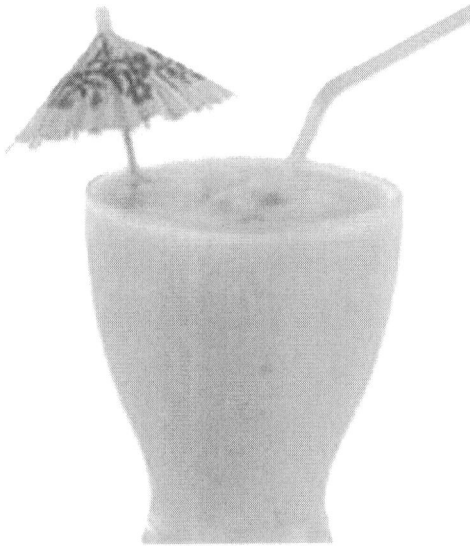

Preparation Time: 5 minutes
Total Time: 5 minutes
Yield: 1 serving

Ingredients
½ cup pineapple, diced
½ medium banana, sliced
2 tablespoons coconut milk
1 teaspoon flaxseeds
coconut water to max line

Method
1.	Combine the pineapple, banana, coconut milk, flaxseeds, and coconut water in the tall glass. Process in the NutriBullet for 10-12 seconds or until becomes smooth.
2.	Pour mixture in a serving glass. Garnish with a small slice of pineapple, if desired.
3.	Serve and enjoy!

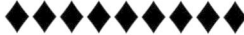

◆◆◆◆◆◆◆◆◆

Orange Carrot and Cucumber Blast

This healthy vegetable drink made with orange, carrot, and cucumber is nice to have for breakfast or snack. It is packed with fiber, antioxidants, vitamins, and minerals that promotes heart health.

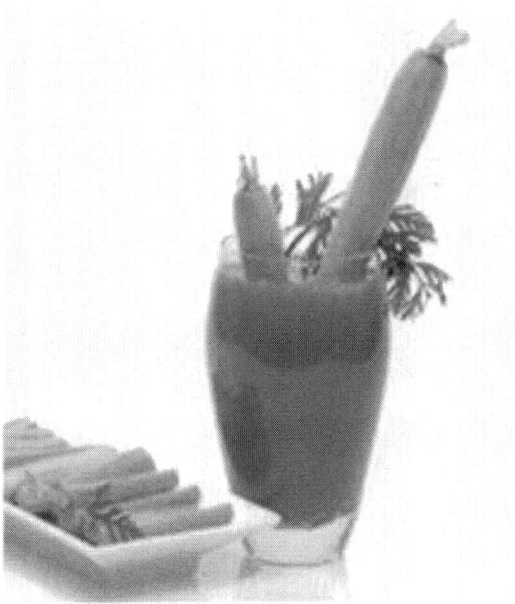

Preparation Time: 5 minutes
Total Time: 5 minutes
Yield: 1 serving

Ingredients

½ medium carrot, diced
½ medium cucumber, diced
½ cup freshly squeezed orange juice
1 teaspoon honey
water to max line

Method

1.　　In the tall glass, place the carrot, cucumber, orange juice, honey, and water. Process in the NutriBullet for 20 seconds or until becomes smooth.
2.　　Pour mixture in a serving glass. Garnish with a slice of orange or small carrot, if desired.
3.　　Serve and enjoy!

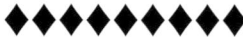

◆◆◆◆◆◆◆◆◆

Watermelon Hemp and Soy Yogurt Cooler

This wonderful smoothie made with watermelon, hemp seeds, and soy yogurt contains good amounts of fiber and antioxidants that can help lower cholesterol levels.

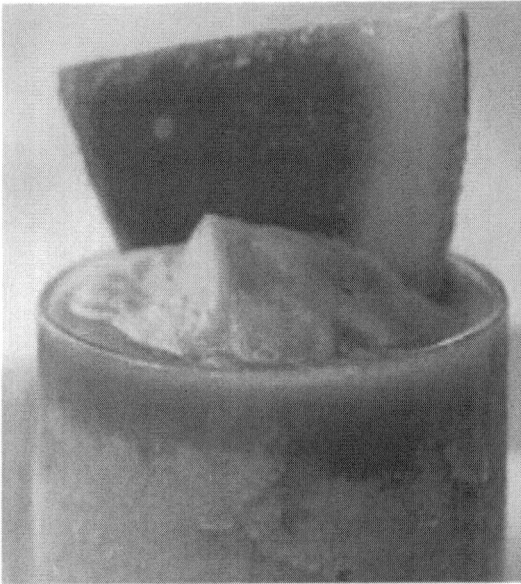

Preparation Time: 5 minutes
Total Time: 5 minutes
Yield: 1 serving

Ingredients

¾ cup seedless watermelon, cubed
½ cup soy yogurt
1 teaspoon hemp seeds
½ cup crushed ice

Method

1.   Place watermelon, yogurt, hemp seeds, and crushed ice in the tall glass. Process in the NutriBullet for 10-12 seconds or until smooth and creamy.
2.   Pour mixture in a chilled glass. Garnish with small slice of watermelon, if desired.
3.   Serve and enjoy!

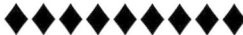

◆◆◆◆◆◆◆◆◆

Cinnamon Apple and Lettuce Smoothie

This amazing smoothie recipe with cinnamon, apple, and lettuce makes a great snack for those people who wants some twist to their regular smoothie.

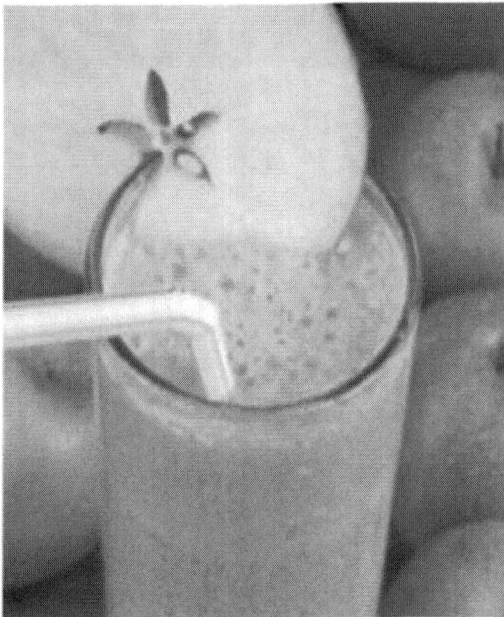

Preparation Time: 5 minutes
Total Time: 5 minutes
Yield: 1 serving

Ingredients
1 handful Romaine lettuce
½ teaspoon cinnamon, ground
1 medium green apple, cored and sliced
¾ cup Greek yogurt, vanilla
water to max line

Method
1.   Combine lettuce, cinnamon, green apple, Greek yogurt, and water in the tall glass. Process in the NutriBullet for 10-15 seconds or until becomes smooth.
2.   Pour in a serving glass. Garnish with apple slices, if desired.
3.   Serve and enjoy!

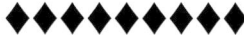

◆◆◆◆◆◆◆◆◆

Blackberry Fennel and Lime Blast with Honey

This low calorie drink with blackberries, fennel, lime, and honey is great for those who want to have a healthy and delicious beverage to pair with their hearty meals.

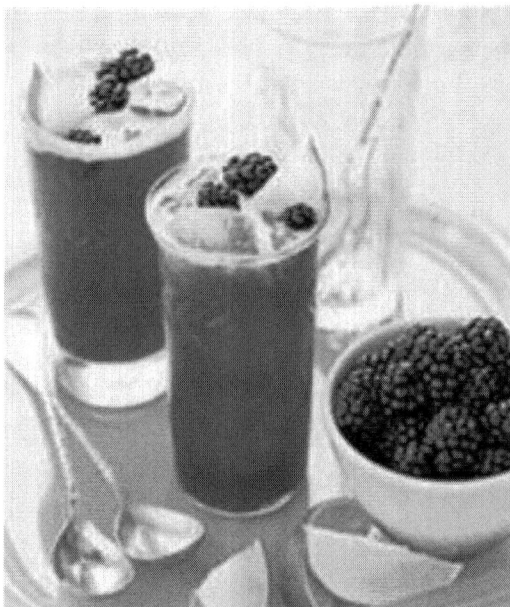

Preparation Time: 5 minutes
Total Time: 5 minutes
Yield: 1 serving

Ingredients
¾ cup blackberries
¼ medium fennel bulb, shredded
1 tablespoon lime juice
1 teaspoon honey
water to max line
ice cubes, to serve

Method
1.   Place blackberries, fennel, lime juice, honey, and water in the tall glass. Process in the NutriBullet for 10-15 seconds or until combined well.
2.   Pour in a serving glass over ice cubes. Garnish with a few blackberries, if desired.
3.   Serve and enjoy!

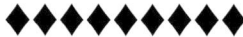

◆◆◆◆◆◆◆◆◆

Kiwi Banana and AvocadoBlast with Chia

This smoothie recipe with kiwi, banana, avocado, and chia will help lift your energy level and sustain you throughout the day because it contains high amount of fiber and healthy kind of fats.

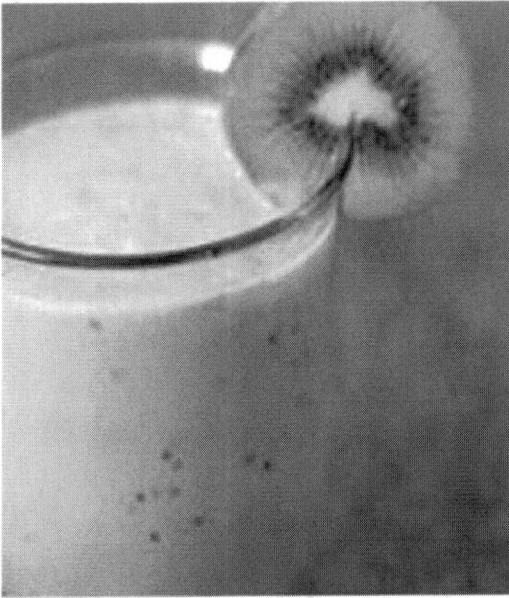

Preparation Time: 5 minutes
Total Time: 5 minutes
Yield: 1 serving

Ingredients
1 medium kiwi, diced
¼ medium avocado, diced
½ cup skim milk
1 teaspoon honey
1 teaspoon chia seeds
water to max line

Method
1.	Place kiwi, avocado, skim milk, honey, chia seeds, and water into the tall glass. Puree in the NutriBullet for 10-15 seconds or until becomes smooth.
2.	Pour in a chilled serving glass. Garnish with a slice of kiwi, if desired.
3.	Serve and enjoy!

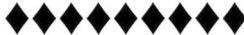

◆◆◆◆◆◆◆◆◆

Melon Carrot and Almond Smoothie with Pumpkin Seed

If you are in search for a healthy and satisfying beverage for breakfast or afternoon snack this is the perfect recipe for you. This delicious smoothie is made of melon, carrot, and almond milk and pumpkin seeds.

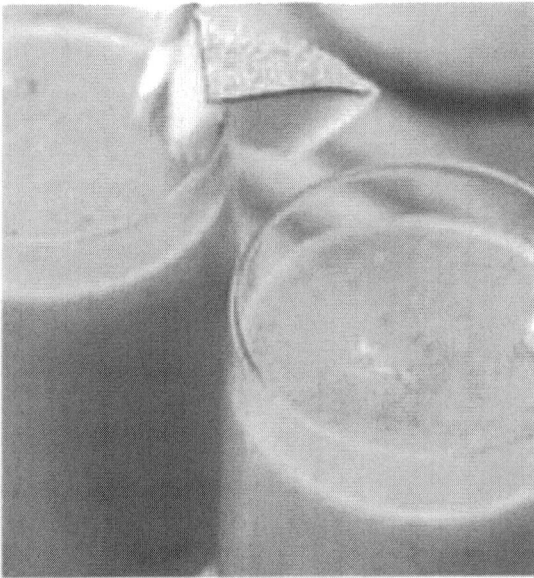

Preparation Time: 5 minutes
Total Time: 5 minutes
Yield:1 serving

Ingredients
¾ cup melon, diced
½ medium carrot, diced
½ cup almond milk
2 Tbsp. pumpkin seeds

Method
1.   Combine melon, carrot, almond milk, and pumpkin seeds in the tall glass. Process in the NutriBullet for 20 seconds or until mixture becomes smooth and creamy.
2.   Pour in a serving glass. Garnish with a small slice of melon, if desired.
3.   Serve and enjoy!

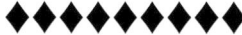

◆◆◆◆◆◆◆◆◆

Watermelon Celery and Fennel Blast

This smoothie recipe with watermelon, celery, and fennel makes a healthy breakfast or snack in a glass!

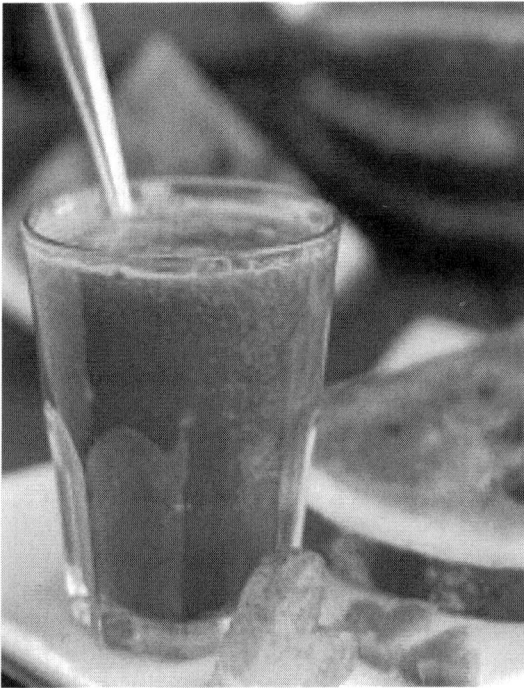

Preparation Time: 5 minutes
Total Time: 5 minutes
Yield: 1 serving

Ingredients
1 cup watermelon, cubed
1 medium celery stalk, diced
½ cup fennel bulb, shredded
1 Tbsp. lime juice
water to max line

Method
1.   Place watermelon, celery, fennel, lime juice, and water in the tall glass. Process in the NutriBullet for 20 seconds or until combined well.
2.   Pour in a serving glass with ice. Garnish with a slice of lime or watermelon, if desired.
3.   Serve and enjoy!

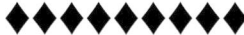

◆◆◆◆◆◆◆◆◆

Blueberry Oat Yogurt and Sunflower Seed Smoothie

This delightful beverage is full of fiber and other properties that promotes healthy heart from the blueberries, oat, yogurt, and sunflower seeds.

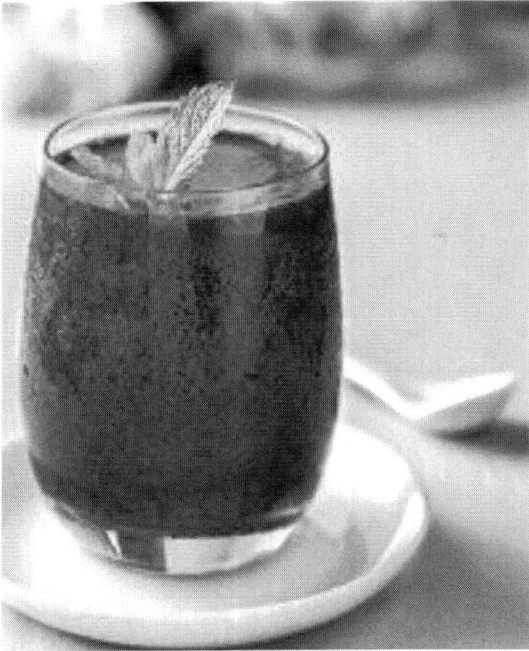

Preparation Time: 5 minutes
Total Time: 5 minutes
Yield:1 serving

Ingredients
½ cup blueberries, frozen
½ cup blackberries, frozen
1 Tbsp. rolled oats
½ cup Greek yogurt, plain or vanilla
1 Tbsp. sunflower seeds

Method
1.   Combine blueberries, blackberries, oats, yogurt, and sunflower seeds in the tall glass. Place and process in the NutriBullet for 10-15 seconds or until smooth.
2.   Pour in a serving glass. Garnish with few berries, if desired.
3.   Serve and enjoy!

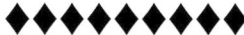

◆◆◆◆◆◆◆◆◆

Berry Soy Yogurt and Pistachio Smoothie

This mouthwatering and refreshing smoothie recipe is made with mixed berries, soy yogurt, soy milk, and pistachios.

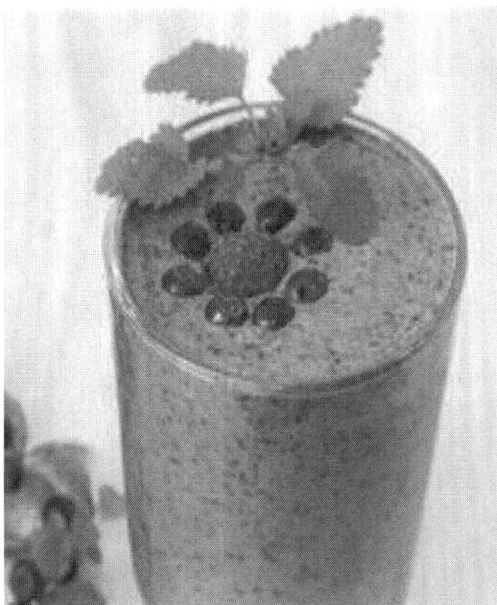

Preparation Time: 5 minutes
Total Time: 5 minutes
Yield: 1 serving

Ingredients

½ cup mixed berries, frozen
¼ cup soy yogurt
½ cup soy milk
6 pistachio nuts

Method

1.   Combine the mixed berries, soy yogurt, soy milk, and pistachios in the tall glass. Process in the NutriBullet for 10-15 seconds or until smooth.

2.   Pour mixture in a serving glass. Garnish with mixed berries, if desired.

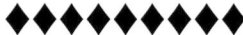

3.   Serve and enjoy!

◆◆◆◆◆◆◆◆

Honeydew Avocado and Almond Smoothie

This delicious and nutritious smoothie recipe is made with honeydew melon, avocado, and almond milk. It is good for you because it is rich in good kind of fats and potassium that promotes heart health.

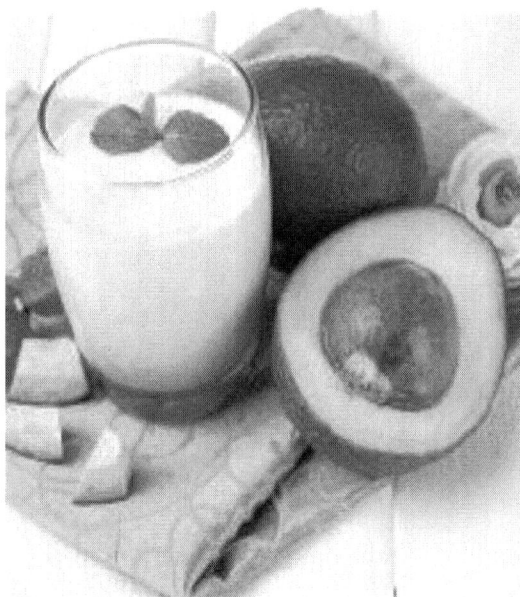

Preparation Time: 5 minutes
Total Time: 5 minutes
Yield: 1 servings

Ingredients
¾ cup honeydew melon, cubed
1/8 medium avocado
¾ cup almond milk
1 Tbsp. lime juice
water to max line

Method
1.   Combine the honeydew melon, avocado, almond milk, lime juice, and water in the tall glass. Process in the NutriBullet for 10-15 seconds or until it becomes smooth.
2.   Pour mixture in a serving glass. Garnish with a small slice of melon or avocado, if desired.
3.   Serve and enjoy!

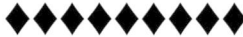

◆◆◆◆◆◆◆◆

Cranberry Banana and Lettuce Smoothie

This is a wonderful beverage recipe made with cranberries, banana, iceberg lettuce and coconut water. If you want to try something new that will give you loads of amazing health benefits this is the recipe for you.

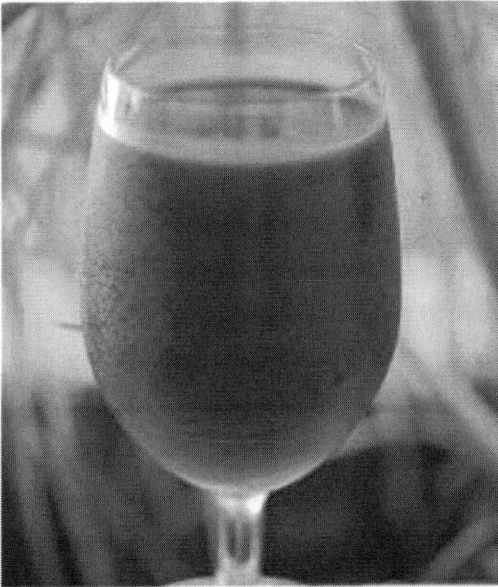

Preparation Time: 5 minutes
Total Time: 5 minutes
Yield: 1 serving
Ingredients

½ cup cranberries
1 medium banana
2 iceberg lettuce leaves, shredded
2/3 cup coconut water
1-2 ice cubes

Method

1.   Combine the cranberries, banana, lettuce, coconut water, and ice cubes in the tall glass. Process in the NutriBullet for 20-30 seconds or until mixture becomes smooth.

2.   Transfer mixture in a serving glass with ice. Garnish with a few cranberries, if desired.

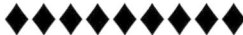

3.   Serve and enjoy!

♦♦♦♦♦♦♦♦♦

Watermelon Yogurt and Oat Blast

This wonderful pink smoothie recipe is packed with dietary fiber and healthy fats from the watermelon, yogurt and oats. A great tasting meal on the go.

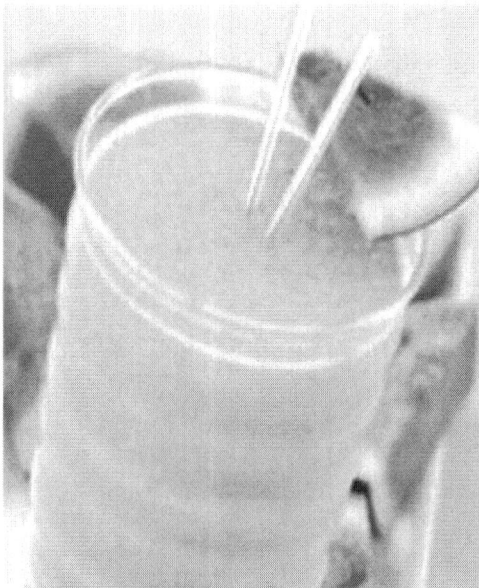

Preparation Time: 5 minutes
Total Time: 5 minutes
Yield: 1 serving

Ingredients

¾ cup watermelon, cut into small pieces
½ cup low-fat yogurt, plain or vanilla
2 tablespoons rolled oats
1 tablespoon wheat germ
water to max line

Method

1.   Combine watermelon, yogurt, oats, wheat germ, and water in the tall glass. Place and process in the NutriBullet for 10-15 seconds or until smooth.
2.   Pour in a serving glass. Garnish with watermelon slices, if desired.
3.   Serve and enjoy!

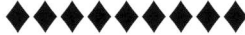

♦♦♦♦♦♦♦♦♦

Apple Avocado Duet with Chia Seeds

This smoothie recipe with apple, avocado, and chia seeds makes a great snack or breakfast on the go because it has generous amount of nutrients for you to stay strong and healthy.

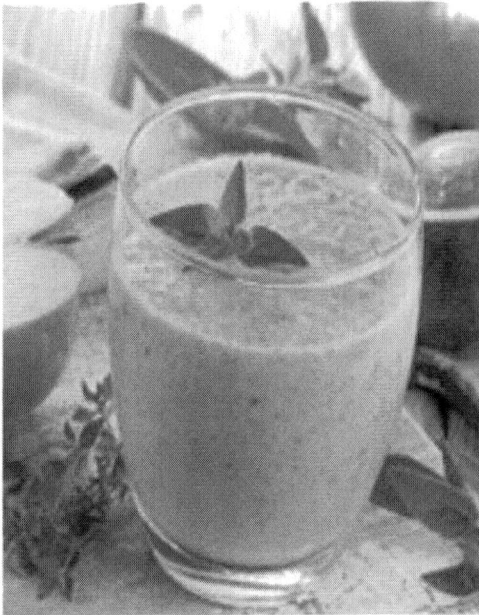

Preparation Time: 5 minutes
Total Time: 5 minutes
Yield: 1 serving

Ingredients

1 medium apple, cored and diced
1/8 medium avocado, diced
¾ cup skim milk
1 teaspoon chia seeds

Method

1.   Place apple, avocado, skim milk, and chia seeds into the tall glass. Puree in the NutriBullet for 10-15 seconds or until becomes smooth.
2.   Pour in a chilled serving glass.
3.   Serve and enjoy!

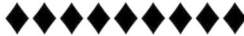

Pineapple Avocado and Parsley Smoothie

This delicious green smoothie recipe made with pineapple, avocado, and parsley is rich in fiber, vitamins and minerals which promotes overall wellness.

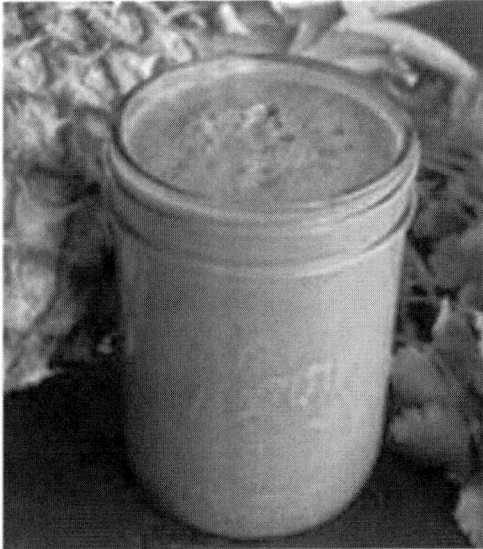

Preparation Time: 5 minutes
Total Time: 5 minutes
Yield: 1 serving

Ingredients

1 cup pineapple, cubed
1/8 medium avocado, diced
1 handful flat-leaf parsley, coarsely chopped
water to max line

Method

1.   Combine pineapple, avocado, parsley, and water in the tall glass. Process in the NutriBullet for 20 seconds or until smooth.
2.   Pour mixture in a serving glass. Garnish with a small chunk of pineapple or fresh parsley, if desired.
3.   Serve and enjoy!

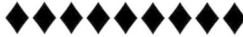

◆◆◆◆◆◆◆◆◆

Ginger Spiced Beet Smoothie with Flax Seeds

This mildly spiced smoothie recipe made with beet root, ginger, and flax seeds is a beverage full of nutrients that are good for you.

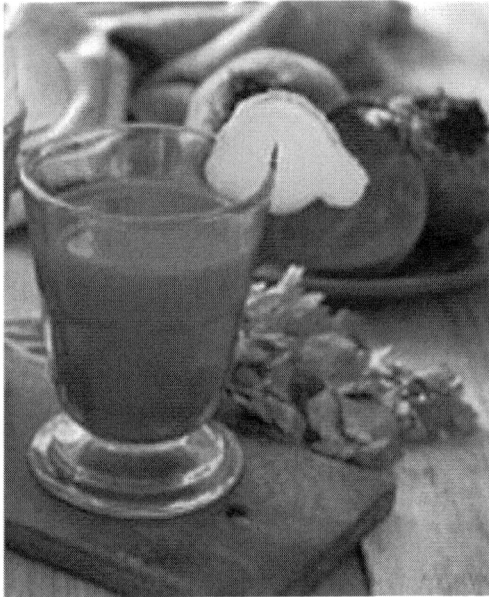

Preparation Time: 5 minutes
Total Time: 5 minutes
Yield: 1 serving

Ingredients

1 medium beet root, diced
½ teaspoon fresh ginger, grated
1 teaspoon flax seeds
coconut water to max line

Method

1.	Place the beet root, coconut water, ginger, flax seeds, and water in the tall glass. Process in the NutriBullet for 10-15 seconds or until smooth.

2.	Pour mixture in a serving glass. Garnish with a thin slice of ginger, if desired.

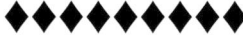

3.	Serve and enjoy!

◆◆◆◆◆◆◆◆◆

Melon Yogurt and Ginger Smoothie

This is a nutrition packed drink that you can have for a quick snack. It is made with melon, ginger, yogurt, and coconut water. Ginger is added to give you more health benefits.

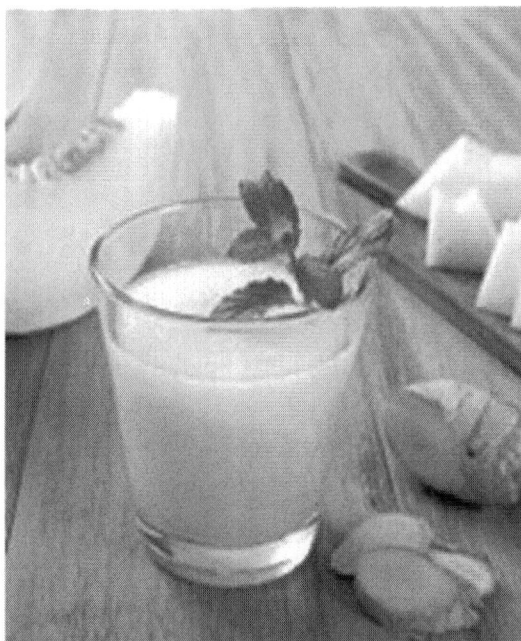

Preparation Time: 5 minutes
Total Time: 5 minutes
Yield: 1 serving

Ingredients
¾ cup cantaloupe melon
½ cup low-fat yogurt
½ teaspoon ginger, grated
coconut water to max line

Method
1.   In the tall glass, place the cantaloupe, low-fat yogurt, ginger, and coconut water. Process in the NutriBullet for 20 seconds or until becomes smooth.
2.   Pour mixture in a serving glass. Garnish with a slice of ginger, if desired.
3.   Serve and enjoy!

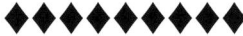

◆◆◆◆◆◆◆◆

Avocado Cucumber Almond and Honey Shake

This super awesome avocado smoothie recipe made with cucumber, walnut, almond milk, and honey will surely brighten up your day.

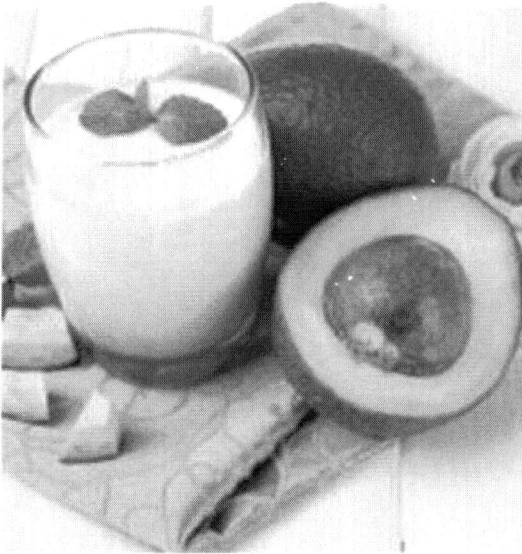

Preparation Time: 5 minutes
Total Time: 5 minutes
Yield:1 serving

Ingredients

1/8 medium avocado, diced
1/3 medium cucumber, diced
¾ cup almond milk

1 teaspoon honey
1-2 ice cubes

Method

1.   Combine avocado, cucumber, almond milk, honey, and ice cubes in the tall glass. Process in the NutriBullet for 20-30 seconds or until mixture becomes smooth.
2.   Pour in a serving glass. Garnish with a slice of avocado, if desired.
3.   Serve and enjoy!

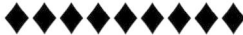

◆◆◆◆◆◆◆◆◆

Minty Banana Apple and Yogurt Smoothie

This awesome smoothie with banana, apple, yogurt, and mint can give you loads of nutrition and a cool feeling especially when taken during hot weather.

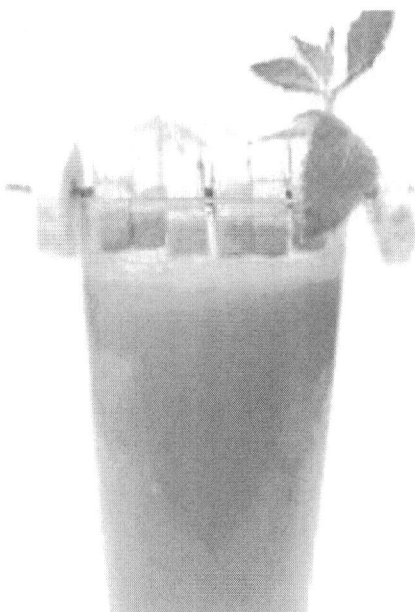

Preparation Time: 5 minutes
Total Time: 5 minutes
Yield: 1 serving

Ingredients
1 medium banana, cut into small pieces
½ mediumapple, cored and iced
½ cup Greek yogurt
1 mint sprig
water to max line

Method
1.   Place banana, apple, yogurt, mint, and water in the tall glass. Process in the NutriBullet for 20 seconds or until it becomes smooth.
2.   Pour in a chilled serving glass. Garnish with banana slices and mint, if desired.
3.   Serve and enjoy!

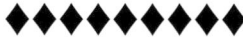

◆◆◆◆◆◆◆◆◆

Minty Mango Soy Smoothie with Chia

This lactose-free smoothie recipe with mango, soy milk, mint, and chia seeds is best to have for a quick breakfast or before and after workout snack.

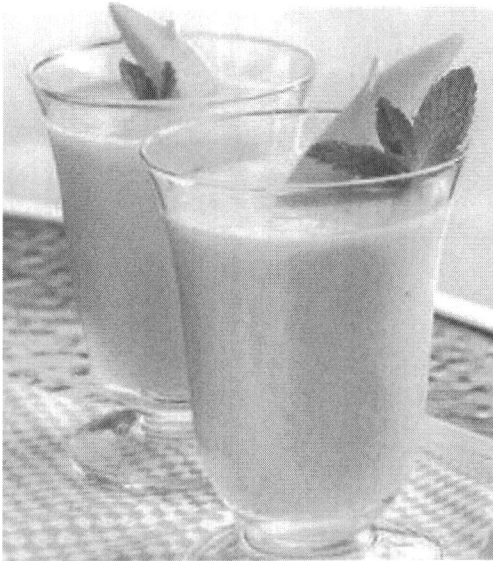

Preparation Time: 5 minutes
Total Time: 5 minutes
Yield: 1 serving

Ingredients

¾ cup mango, sliced
¾ cup soy milk

1 teaspoon chia seeds
1 fresh mint sprig
1-2 ice cubes

Method

1.   Combine mango, soy milk, chia seeds, mint, and ice cubes in the tall glass. Process in the NutriBullet for 20-30 seconds or until it becomes smooth.
2.   Pour in a serving glass. Garnish with a small slice of mango and mint sprig, if desired.
3.   Serve and enjoy!

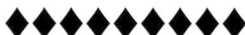

◆◆◆◆◆◆◆◆◆

Minty Strawberry Avocado Soy Smoothie

This a cool and refreshing beverage made with strawberry, avocado, soy milk and mint. This is a nice drink to have especially the weather is hot. It contains healthy fats from avocados and antioxidants from strawberries and soya.

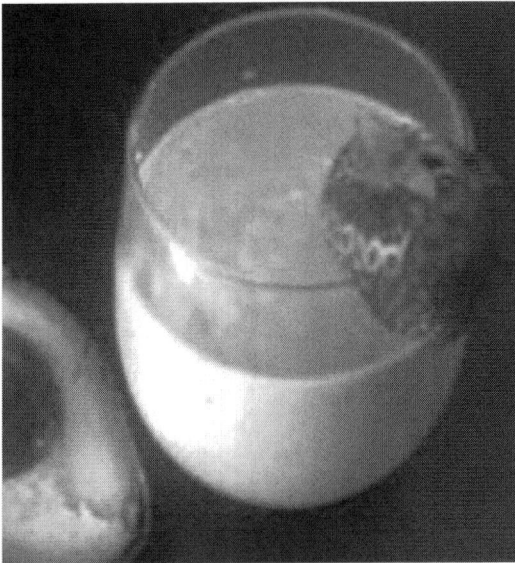

Preparation Time: 5 minutes
Total Time: 5 minutes
Yield:1 serving

Ingredients

½ cup strawberries, halved
1/8medium avocado, sliced
1 cup soy milk, vanilla
1 fresh mint sprig

Method

1.   Combine strawberries, avocado, soy milk, and mint in the tall glass. Place and process in the NutriBullet for 20 seconds or until becomes smooth.

2.   Pour in a serving glass. Garnish with a small strawberry and mint sprig, if desired.

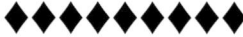

3.   Serve and enjoy!

◆◆◆◆◆◆◆◆

Pistachio and Kale Smoothie

You gotta love pistachio – this delicate, earthy and rich nut that creates fabulous drinks and desserts. This particular recipe offers you a drink that has a bright color and a rich taste and it is perfect for an early morning drink to brighten up your day and awaken your senses.

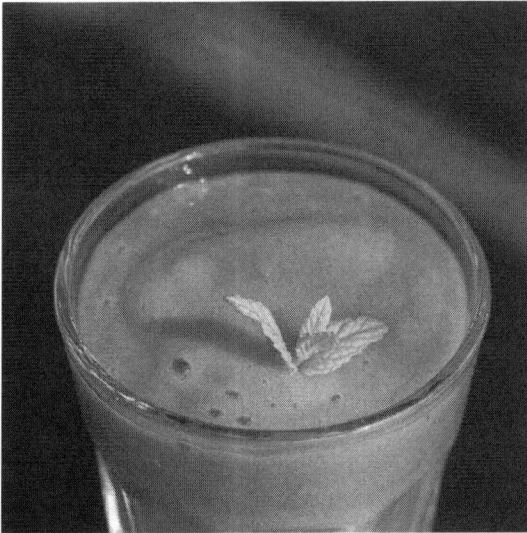

Preparation Time: 5 minutes
Total Time: 5 minutes
Yield: 1 serving

Ingredients
2 kale leaves

¼ cup pistachio nuts
¼ cup plain yogurt
½ cup almond milk
½ teaspoon vanilla extract
1 teaspoon honey
1-2 ice cubes

Method

1.   Combine kale leaves, pistachio, yogurt, almondmilk, vanilla extract, honey and ice in the tall glass. Process in the NutriBullet for 20-30 seconds or until mixture becomes smooth.
2.   Transfer mixture in a serving glass.
3.   Serve and enjoy!

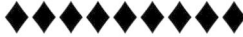

◆◆◆◆◆◆◆◆◆

Pomegranate Spinach and Flax Smoothie

I highly recommend combining fruits with veggies if you are aiming for healthy and nutritious drinks. And from all the veggies available, spinach is definitely one of the easiest to pair with fruits because it is fairly mild in terms of taste, but high in nutrients.

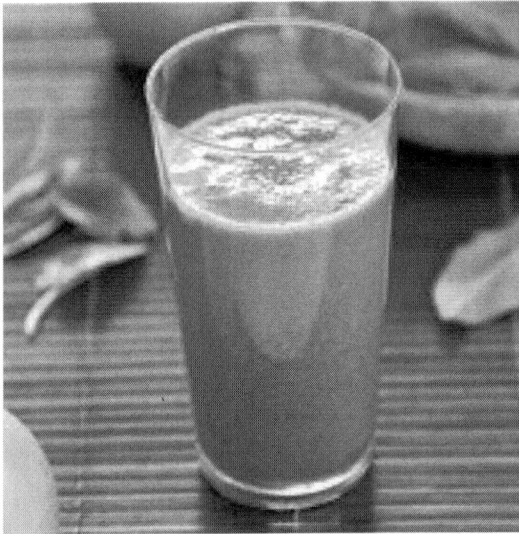

Preparation Time: 5 minutes
Total Time: 5 minutes
Yield:1 serving

Ingredients

1 handful fresh spinach
½ cup pomegranate juice
1 small banana
¼ cup plain yogurt
1 teaspoon agave syrup or honey
1 tablespoon flax seeds
Water to max line

Method

1.　　Combine spinach, pomegranate juice, banana, yogurt, agave syrup or honey, flaxseeds and water in the tall glass. Process in the NutriBullet for 10-15 seconds or until mixture becomes smooth.

2.　　Transfer mixture in a serving glass.

3.　　Serve and enjoy!

◆◆◆◆◆◆◆◆◆

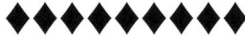

Raspberry Apple Lettuce Smoothie

This awesome smoothie with raspberries, apple, lettuce and skim milk can definitely give you the boost you need to fight diseases or infections caused by free radicals because this drink has high amounts of antioxidants.

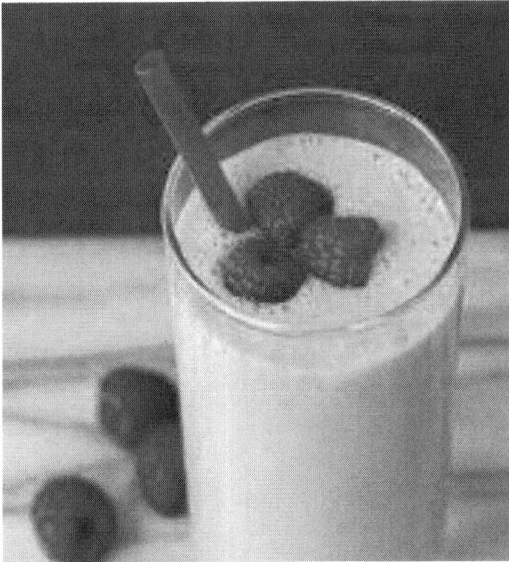

Preparation Time: 5 minutes
Total Time: 5 minutes
Yield: 1 serving

Ingredients

½ cup frozen raspberries
1 small red apple, peeled, cored, cut into small pieces
2 pieces lettuce leaves, torn
¾ cup skim milk

Method

1.   Place raspberries, apple, lettuce, and skim milk in the tall glass. Process in

the NutriBullet for 10-15 seconds or until becomes smooth and creamy.

2.   Pour in a chilled serving glass. Garnish with raspberries, if desired.

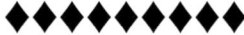

3.   Serve and enjoy!

◆◆◆◆◆◆◆◆◆

Raspberry Dates and Sunflower Seeds Smoothie

This is such a refreshing smoothie, the raspberries blends perfect with dates and sunflower seeds. It is rich in antioxidants that are good for the heart.

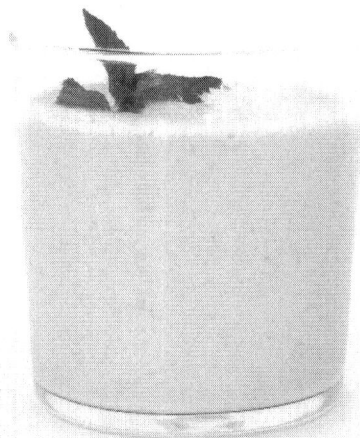

Preparation Time: 5 minutes
Total Time: 5 minutes
Yield:1 serving

Ingredients
½ cup fresh raspberries
2 dates, pitted
2/3 cup skim milk
½ cup plain yogurt
2 tablespoonssunflower seeds

Method
1.   Combine dates, raspberries, skim milk, yogurt, and sunflower seeds in the tall glass. Process in the NutriBullet for

10-15 seconds or until mixture becomes smooth.
2.   Transfer mixture in a serving glass.
3.   Serve and enjoy!

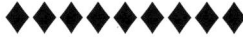

◆◆◆◆◆◆◆◆◆

Raspberry Papaya and Coconut Smoothie

This smoothie has the taste of the tropics. You will love the combination of the raspberries,papaya, and coconut. They come together in this delicious and nutritious drink.

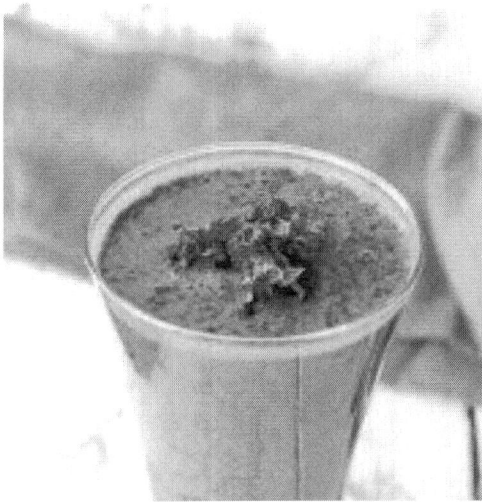

Preparation Time: 5 minutes
Total Time: 5 minutes
Yield:1 serving

Ingredients
½ cup fresh raspberries
¾ cup papaya, peeled
2 tablespoon rolled oats
2 Tbsp. coconut milk
1 teaspoon agave syrup (optional)
coconut water to max line

Method
1.   Combine raspberries, papaya, rolled oats, coconut milk, agave syrup, and coconut water in the tall glass.

Process in the NutriBullet for 20 seconds
or until mixture becomes smooth.

2.   Transfer mixture in a serving glass.

3.   Serve and enjoy!

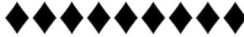

Walnut Raspberry and Banana Shake

This power-packed smoothie recipe with walnuts, raspberries and banana is the perfect beverage for busy days when you don't have much time to prepare a hearty meal.

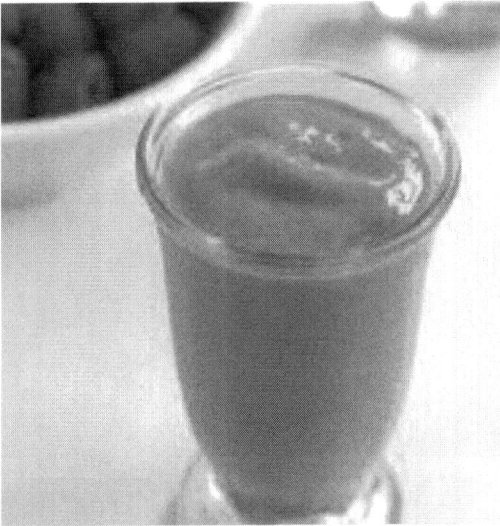

Preparation Time: 5 minutes
Total Time: 5 minutes
Yield: 1 serving

Ingredients

3/4 cup raspberries, halved
½ medium banana, cut into small pieces

6 pcs. walnuts
2/3 cup skim milk

Method

1.   Place the raspberries, banana, walnuts, and skim milk in the tall glass. Process in the NutriBullet for 10-15 seconds or until it becomes smooth.
2.   Pour in a chilled tall glass. Garnish with raspberries, if desired.
3.   Serve and enjoy!

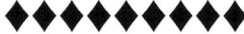

◆◆◆◆◆◆◆◆◆

Watermelon and Basil Smoothie

This combination sounds unusual, but I promise that it works great. The fresh watermelon tones down the basil which only adds a touch of aroma without becoming overpowering. This drink is certified delicious and also nutritious.

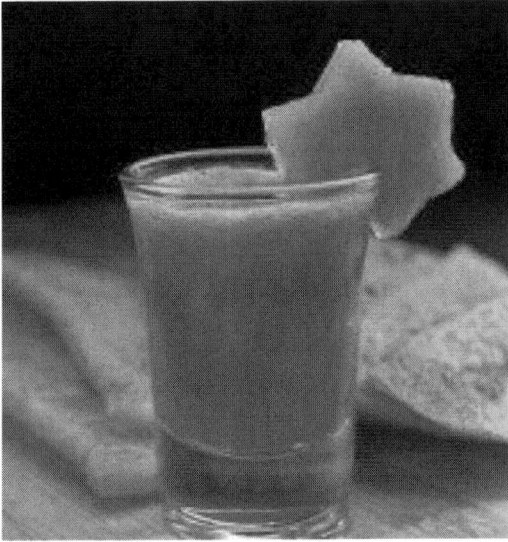

Preparation Time: 5 minutes
Total Time: 5 minutes
Yield:1 serving

Ingredients
1 cup seedless watermelon cubes
2-3 basil leaves
1 Tbsp. lime juice
1 tsp. honey
1-2 ice cubes
water to max line

Method
1.   Combine watermelon, basil leaves, lime juice, honey, ice cubes, and water in

the tall glass. Process in the NutriBullet for 20-30 seconds or until mixture becomes smooth.

2.   Transfer mixture in a serving glass.

3.   Serve and enjoy!

♦♦♦♦♦♦♦♦♦

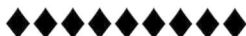

Watermelon Lemonade

Yes, you can make lemonade in your Nutribullet and not just any lemonade, but a watermelon one – nutritious, delicious, refreshing and light.

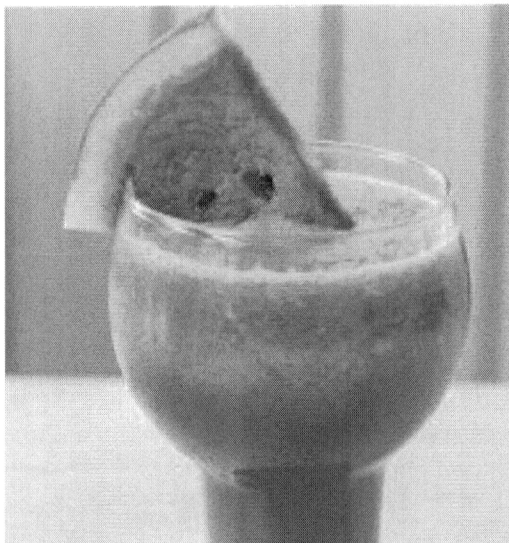

Preparation Time: 5 minutes
Total Time: 5 minutes
Yield:1 serving

Ingredients
1 cup seedless watermelon cubes
2 tablespoon lemon juice
½ cup sparkling water
2-3 ice cubes
1 teaspoon honey

Method
1.   Combine watermelon, lemon juice, sparkling water, ice and honey in the tall glass. Process in the NutriBullet for 20-30

seconds or until mixture becomes smooth.

2.   Transfer mixture in a serving glass.
3.   Serve and enjoy!

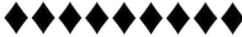

♦♦♦♦♦♦♦♦♦

Banana Peach and Nutmeg Smoothie

The nice sweet flavor of peach combines well with the creaminessof banana, creating a drink that tastes amazing and is loaded with nutrients.

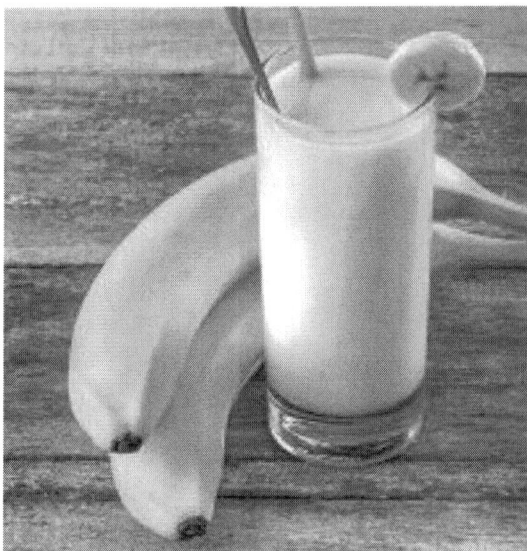

Preparation Time: 5minutes
Total Time: 5 minutes
Yield:1 serving

Ingredients
1 small ripe banana, cut into small pieces
2 peach halves, diced

¾ cup almond milk
pinch nutmeg
pinch cinnamon

Method
1.   Combine all the ingredients in your Nutribullet and process 20-30 seconds until well blended.
2.   Pour in a serving glass and serve immediately.

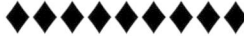

♦♦♦♦♦♦♦♦♦

Spiced Mango Yogurt Smoothie (Mango Lassi)

Lassi is an Indian drink usually made with yogurt and fruits and this mango version really makes this drink shine with its amazing taste.

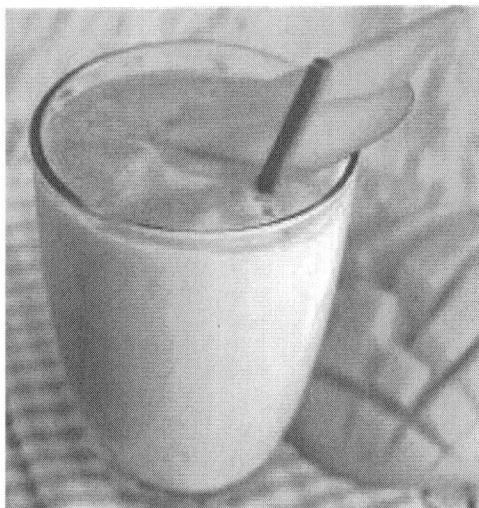

Preparation Time: 5 minutes
Total Time: 5 minutes
Yield: 1 serving

Ingredients

½ cup ripe mango, peeled and cubed
½ cup plain yogurt
¼ cup skim milk
1 teaspoon honey

½ teaspoon fresh ginger, grated
pinch cardamom
1-2 ice cubes

Method

1.   Combine mango, yogurt, milk, honey, ginger, cardamom, and ice cubes in the tall glass. Process in the NutriBullet for 20-30 seconds or until mixture becomes smooth.
2.   Transfer mixture in a serving glass.
3.   Serve and enjoy!

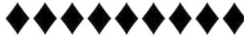

◆◆◆◆◆◆◆◆◆

Melon Lettuce and Almond Smoothie

Don't underestimate the nutrients found in lettuce. You will be surprised to know that lettuce is high in minerals and vitamin C. The melon mellows down the taste of lettuce and the final drink is awesome.

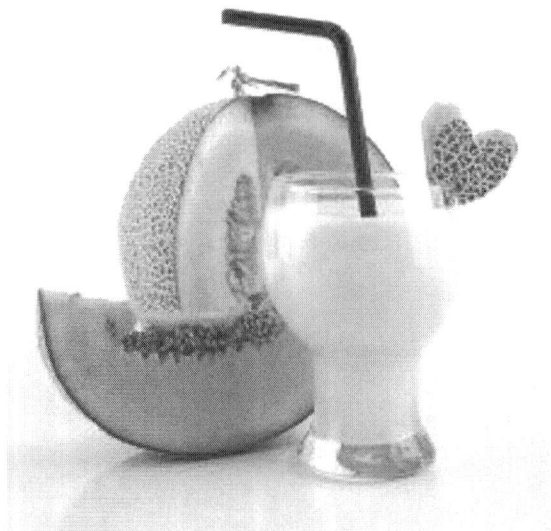

Preparation Time: 5 minutes
Total Time: 5 minutes
Yield:1 serving

Ingredients

1 cup cantaloupe melon, cubed
2 lettuce leaves
½ cup almond milk
1 teaspoon agave nectar

Method

1.   Combine melon, lettuce, almond milk, and agave syrup in the tall glass.

Process in the NutriBullet for 20 seconds
or until mixture becomes smooth.
2.   Transfer mixture in a serving glass.
3.   Serve and enjoy!

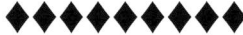

◆◆◆◆◆◆◆◆◆

Banana Yogurt Smoothie
with Pumpkin Seeds

*Nothing tastes better than this delicious
summer smoothie! Just what you need
during those hot summer days.*

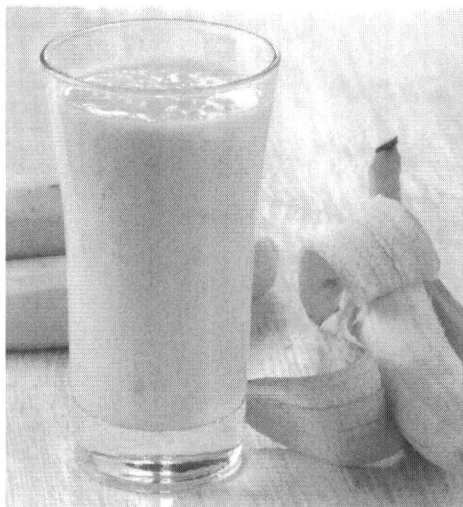

Preparation Time: 5 minutes
Total Time: 5 minutes
Yield:1 serving

Ingredients

1 medium banana, cut into small pieces
½ cup Greek yogurt, vanilla
2/3 cup almond milk
2 tablespoonspumpkin seeds
1-2 ice cubes

Method

1.   Combine banana, yogurt, almond milk, pumpkin seeds, and ice cubes in the tall glass. Process in the NutriBullet for

20-30 seconds or until mixture becomes smooth.

2.   Transfer mixture in a serving glass.

3.   Serve and enjoy!

♦♦♦♦♦♦♦♦

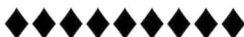

Minty Cantaloupe Chilled Smoothie

Cantaloupe melon tastes amazing and at the same time nutritious. It's a simple drink that relies on the great combination of cantaloupe, yogurt and almond milk with a hint of mint.

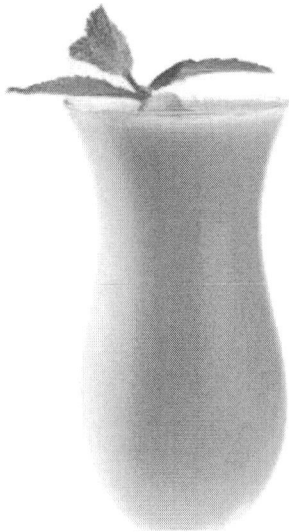

Preparation Time: 5 minutes
Total Time: 5 minutes
Yield:1 serving

Ingredients
¾ cup cantaloupe cubes
¼ cup plain yogurt
2/3 cup almond milk
¼ teaspoon vanilla extract
1 mint sprig
1-2 ice cubes

Method
1.   Combine cantaloupe, yogurt, almond milk, vanilla extract, mint, and ice

in the tall glass. Process in the NutriBullet for 20-30 seconds or until mixture becomes smooth.

2.   Transfer mixture in a serving glass.

3.   Serve and enjoy!

♦♦♦♦♦♦♦♦♦

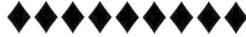

Orange and Carrot Super Healthy Smoothie

Both orange and carrotare rich sources of antioxidants that are beneficial for keeping our body cells healthy.

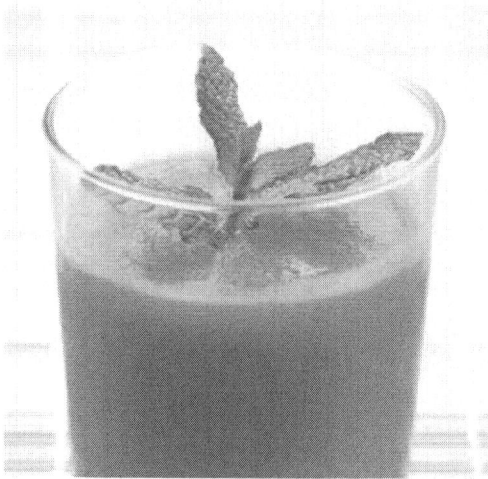

Preparation Time: 5 minutes
Total Time: 5 minutes
Yield:1 serving

Ingredients
1 medium orange, cut into segments
1 small carrot, sliced
1 teaspoon orange zest, grated
2/3 cup vanilla yogurt
1-2 ice cubes
water to max line

Method
1.   Combine carrot, orange, orange zest, yogurt, ice, and water in the tall glass. Process in the NutriBullet for 20-30 seconds or until mixture becomes smooth.
2.   Transfer mixture in a serving glass.
3.   Serve and enjoy!

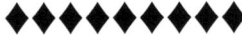

◆◆◆◆◆◆◆◆◆

Pineapple Super Healthy Smoothie

Pineapple is a great source of fiber that can help regulate blood cholesterol levels. Thus, keeping your heart healthy. Plus, it is delicious and makes an excellent drink.

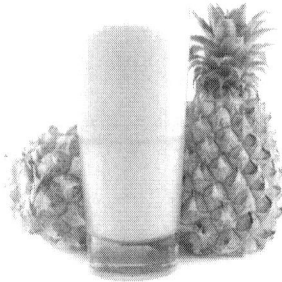

Preparation Time: 5 minutes
Total Time: 5 minutes
Yield: 1 serving

Ingredients

1 cup fresh pineapple, cubed
½ cup plain or vanilla yogurt
½ cup almond milk
1 tablespoon chia seeds

Method

1.   Combine fresh pineapple, yogurt, almond milk, and chia seeds in the tall glass. Process in the NutriBullet for 20 seconds or until mixture becomes smooth.
2.   Transfer mixture in a serving glass.
3.   Serve and enjoy!

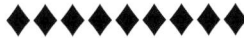

◆◆◆◆◆◆◆◆◆

Spinach and Banana Smoothie

Thick and nutritious, this smoothie is exactly what you need to boost your energy after a long day at work or to jumpstart your mornings.

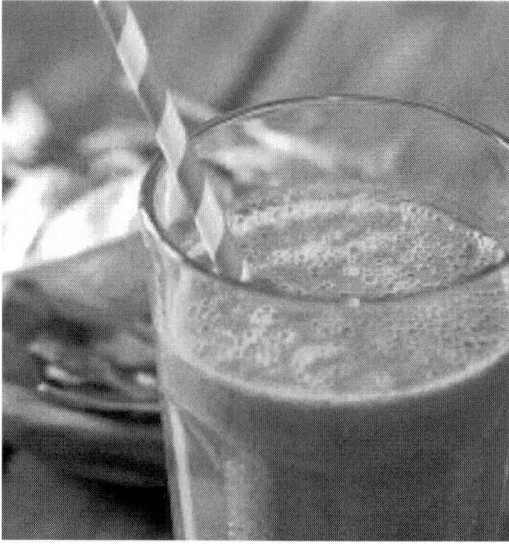

Preparation Time: 5 minutes
Total Time: 5 minutes
Yield:1 serving

Ingredients
1 handful baby spinach
1 medium banana
¾ cup almond milk
¼ cup crushed ice
2 tablespoon wheat germ

Method
1.   Combine spinach, banana, almond milk, ice, and wheat germ the tall glass.

Process in the NutriBullet for 20 seconds or until mixture becomes smooth.

2. Transfer mixture in a serving glass.

3. Serve and enjoy!

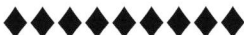

Avocado and Golden Raisin Smoothie

Both raisins and avocado are easy to find all year around and both of them are nutritious being high in fiber and good fats. A glass of this smoothie in the morning will keep you feeling full until your next meal.

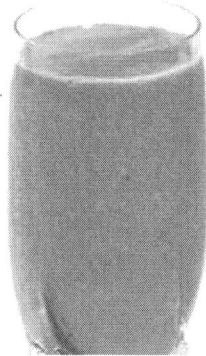

Preparation Time: 5 minutes
Total Time: 5 minutes
Yield: 1 serving

Ingredients
1/8 avocado, diced
¼ cup golden raisins
¾ cup skim milk
1-2 ice cubes

Method

1.   Place avocado, raisins, milk, and ice cubes in the Nutribullet.
2.   Process for 20-30 seconds or until smooth.
3.   Transfer in a serving glass. Enjoy.

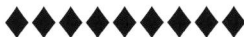

◆◆◆◆◆◆◆◆◆

Autumn Hemp Seed Smoothie

Pumpkin and pear are the main ingredients of this awesome recipe which make this smoothie a real autumn delight, while the hemp seeds boost its nutritional content, creating a filling and nourishing drink for those cold days.

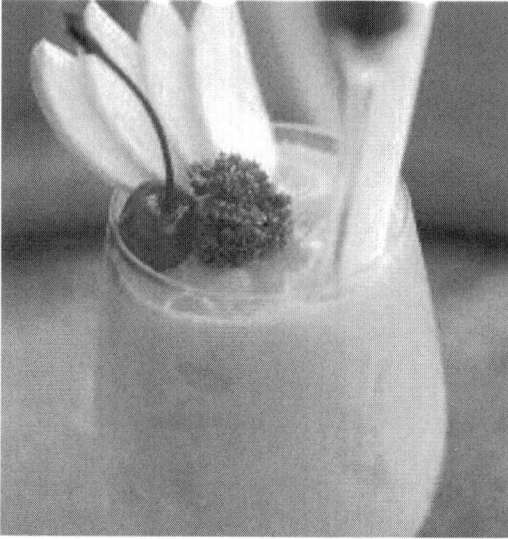

Preparation Time: 5 minutes
Total Time: 5 minutes
Yield:1 serving

Ingredients

½ cup pumpkin puree
1 medium pear, cored and diced
¼ teaspoon fresh ginger, grated
1 teaspoon hemp seeds
½ cup almond milk

Method

1.   Place the pumpkin puree, pear, ginger, hemp seeds, and almond milk in the Nutribullet.

2.   Process for 20 seconds or until smooth.

3.   Transfer in a serving glass. Enjoy.

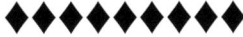

Spinach Sweet Potato and Almond Smoothie

Raw sweet potatoes are an amazing source of nutrients, from fiber to minerals. Plus, they have a rather sweet taste so you don't need to add any other sweetener.

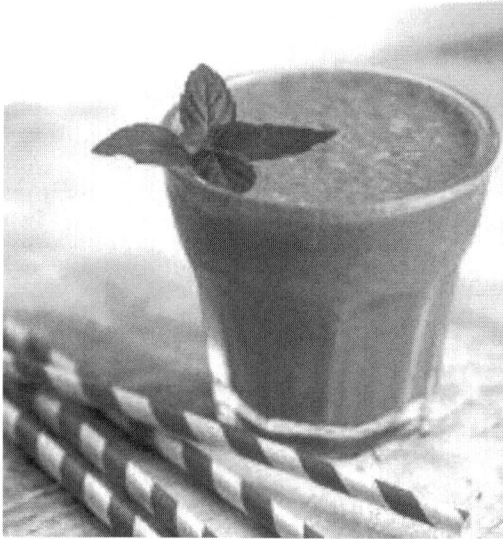

Preparation Time: 5 minutes
Total Time: 5 minutes
Yield: 1 serving

Ingredients

1 medium sweet potato, cubed
1 handful spinach
¾ cup almond milk

1 teaspoon flaxseeds

Method

1.   Combine sweet potato, spinach, almond milk, and flaxseeds in the tall glass. Process in the NutriBullet for 20 seconds or until mixture becomes smooth.
2.   Transfer mixture in a serving glass.
3.   Serve and enjoy!

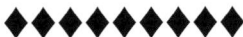

◆◆◆◆◆◆◆◆◆

Raspberry Spinach and Coconut Smoothie

Combining spinach with raspberries and coconut is not unusual for the avid drinkers of healthy smoothies. In fact, it is one of the best combinations you can make because both spinach and strawberries are loaded with much needed nutrients.

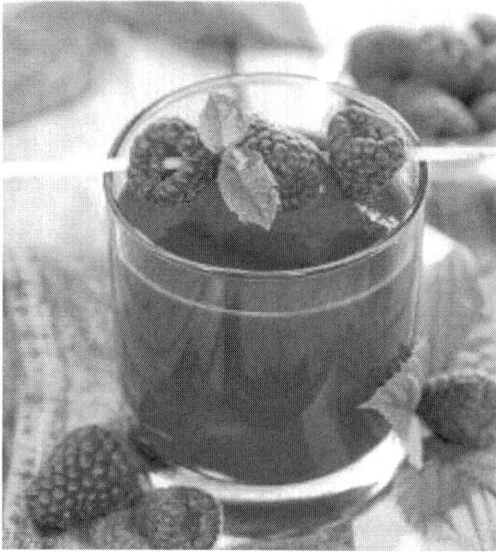

Preparation Time: 5 minutes
Total Time: 5 minutes
Yield: 1 serving

Ingredients

½ cup spinach
½ cup frozen strawberries
2 tablespoons coconut milk
1 teaspoon agave nectar
coconut water to max line

Method

1.   Combine spinach, strawberries, coconut milk, agave syrup, and coconut water in the tall glass. Process in the

NutriBullet for 20 seconds or until mixture becomes smooth.
2.   Transfer mixture in a serving glass.
3.   Serve and enjoy!

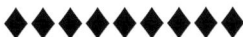

◆◆◆◆◆◆◆◆◆

Watermelon Hemp Seed and Coconut Blast

Don't neglect the health benefits of watermelon. It contains good amounts of fiber, antioxidants, water,vitamins, and minerals which will keep your body hydrated and nourished during those hot summer days.

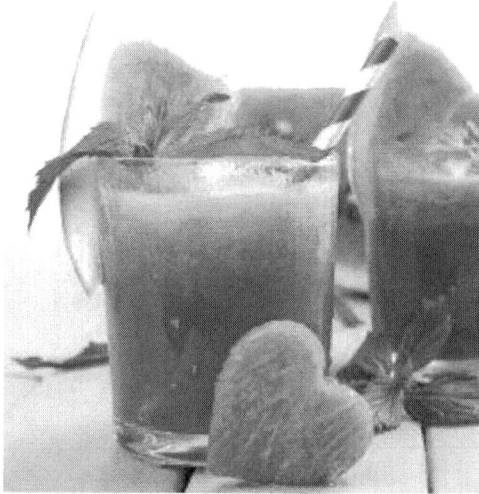

Preparation Time: 5 minutes
Total Time: 5 minutes
Yield:1 serving

Ingredients
1 cup seedless watermelon cubes
2 tsp. hemp seeds
2 ice cubes
coconut water to max line

Method
1.   Combine watermelon, hemp seeds, ice cubes, and coconut water in the tall glass. Process in the NutriBullet for 10-15 seconds or until mixture becomes smooth.

2. Transfer mixture in a serving glass.
3. Serve and enjoy!

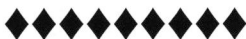

◆◆◆◆◆◆◆◆◆

Kiwi Green Chilled Smoothie

Spinach, kiwi and lemon are the main ingredients of this drink. This is a certified delicious and nutritious summer refreshment that is good for your heart too!

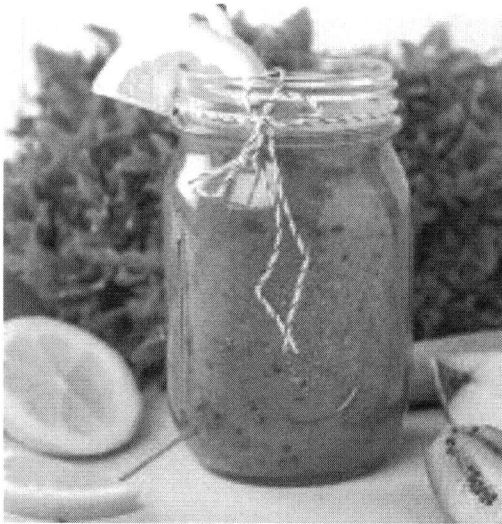

Preparation Time: 5 minutes
Total Time: 5 minutes
Yield: 1 serving

Ingredients
1 kiwi fruit, sliced
1 handful fresh spinach
2 tablespoons lemon juice
1 teaspoon chia seeds

1 teaspoon honey
1-2 ice cubes
coconut water to max line

Method

1.   Combine kiwi, spinach, lemon juice, chia seeds, honey, ice, and coconut water in the tall glass. Process in the NutriBullet for 20 seconds or until mixture becomes smooth.
2.   Transfer mixture in a serving glass.
3.   Serve and enjoy!

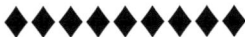

◆◆◆◆◆◆◆◆◆

Grape Apple and Yogurt Smoothie

Both grapes and apples aregreat in terms of nutrients and flavor. You will love this refreshing and light smoothie – it is impressive not only because of its delicious taste, but also its high ability to rehydrate and give you the nutrients you need.

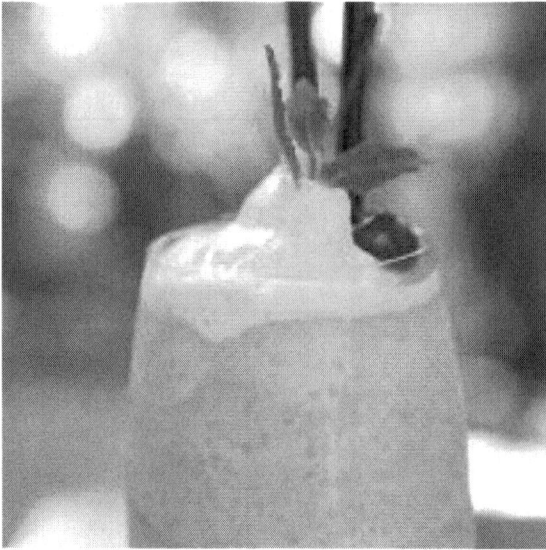

Preparation Time: 5 minutes
Total Time: 5 minutes
Yield:1 serving

Ingredients

½ cup seedless green grapes
1 medium green apple, cored and diced
¾ cup Greek yogurt
¼ cup crushed ice

Method

1.   Combine grapes, apple, yogurt, and ice in the tall glass. Process in the NutriBullet for 20 seconds or until mixture becomes smooth.
2.   Transfer mixture in a serving glass.
3.   Serve and enjoy!

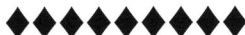

◆◆◆◆◆◆◆◆

Avocado Banana and Orange Smoothie

This delightful smoothie made with avocado, banana, and orange is naturally rich in healthy fats, fiber, vitamins and minerals. These nutrients play a vital role in proper functioning of the body organs like the heart.

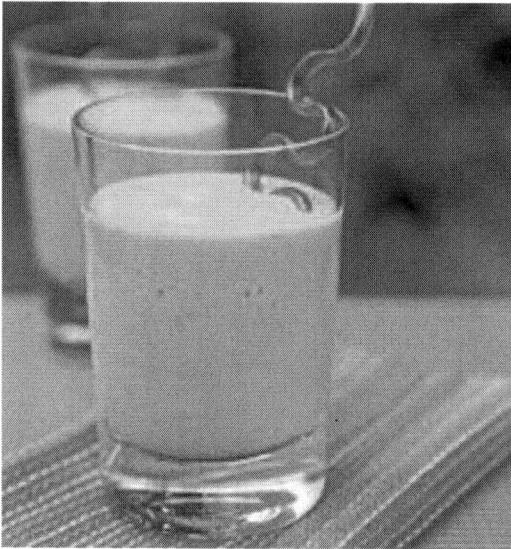

Preparation Time: 5 minutes
Total Time: 5 minutes
Yield:1 serving

Ingredients
¼ medium avocado, diced
1 medium frozen banana, sliced

½ cup fresh orange juice
2 tablespoons rolled oats
water to max line

Method

1.   Place avocado, banana, orange juice, rolled oats, and water in the tall glass. Process in the NutriBullet for 20 seconds or until smooth.

2.   Pour mixture in a chilled glass. Garnish with a slice of orange, if desired.

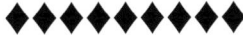

3.   Serve and enjoy!

◆◆◆◆◆◆◆◆◆

Minty Avocado Pineapple and Yogurt Smoothie

A delicious smoothie recipe with avocado, oats, pineapple, mint, and yogurt.

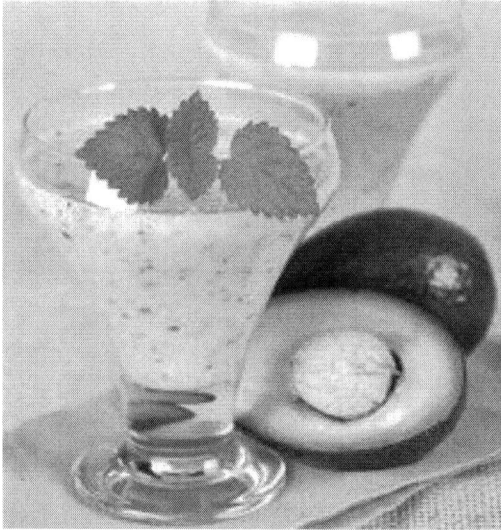

Preparation Time: 5 minutes
Total Time: 5 minutes
Yield: 1 serving

Ingredients

¼ cup ripe avocado, cubed
2 tablespoons rolled oats
½ cup pineapple, cubed
½ cup plain Greek yogurt
1 mint sprig

Method

1.   Combine avocado, rolled oats, pineapple, Greek yogurt, and mint in the tall glass. Process in the NutriBullet for 20 seconds or until mixture becomes smooth.

2.   Transfer mixture in a serving glass. Garnish with mint sprig, if desired.

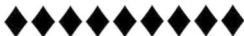

3.   Serve and enjoy!

◆◆◆◆◆◆◆◆

Banana Grape Smoothie Recipe

This awesome smoothie with banana, grapes, and yogurt makes a great tasting and nutritious snack.

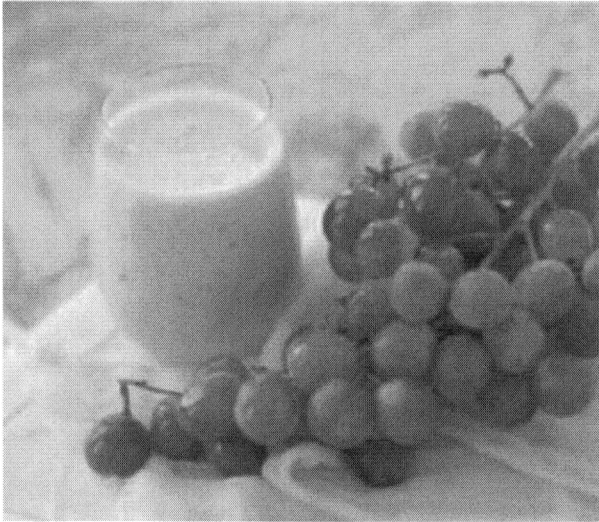

Preparation Time: 5 minutes
Total Time: 5 minutes
Yield:1 serving

Ingredients

1 medium frozen banana, cut into small pieces
12 pieces seedless grapes
½ cup yogurt

water to max line

Method

1.   Place banana, grapes, yogurt, and water in the Nutribullet.
2.   Process for 10-15 seconds or until smooth.
3.   Transfer in a serving glass. Enjoy.

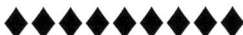

Avocado Spinach and Lemon Smoothie with Honey

This smoothie recipe with avocado, spinach, lemon juice, skim milk, and honey will not only give you energy boost but will also prevent you from many health issues like heart disease.

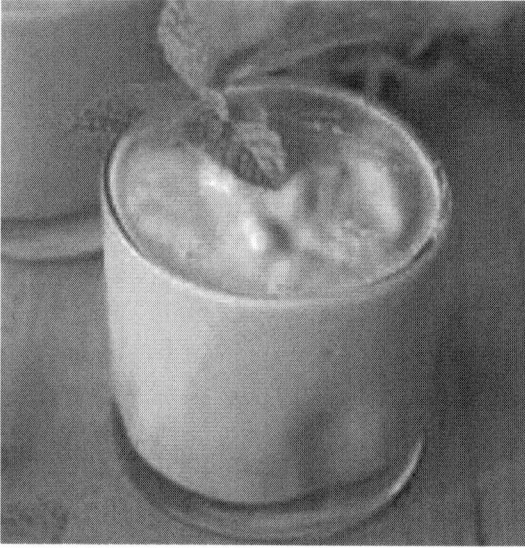

Preparation Time: 5 minutes
Total Time: 5 minutes
Yield: 1 serving

Ingredients

¼ medium avocado
1 cup spinach, torn
1 tablespoon lemon juice

¾ cup skim milk
1 teaspoon honey

Method
1.   Place avocado, spinach, lemon juice, skim milk, and honey into the tall glass. Process in the NutriBullet for 10-15 seconds or until becomes smooth.
2.   Pour in a chilled serving glass. Garnish with a slice of lemon, if desired.
3.   Serve and enjoy!

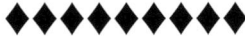

◆◆◆◆◆◆◆◆

Banana Soy Walnut Delight Smoothie

If you are a banana and soy lover, this is the perfect recipe for you. Bananas are naturally rich in fiber and potassium that is good for heart health.

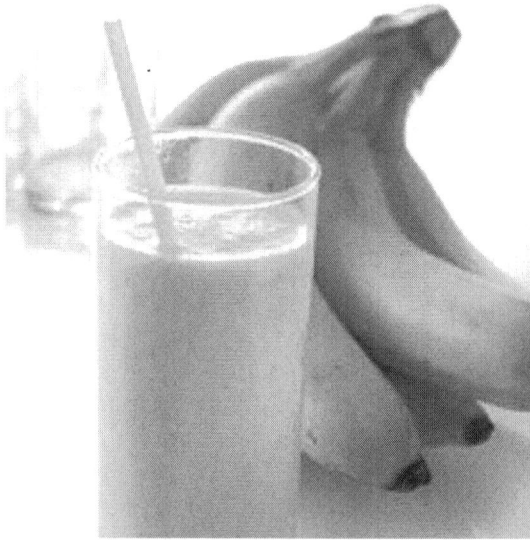

Preparation Time: 5 minutes
Total Time: 5 minutes
Yield: 1 serving

Ingredients

1 medium banana, cut into small pieces
½ cup soy yogurt, vanilla flavour
½ cup soy milk, unsweetened

6 walnuts, coarsely chopped

Method

1.   Combine banana, soy yogurt, soy milk and walnuts in the tall glass. Process in the NutriBullet for 20 seconds or until mixture becomes smooth and creamy.

2.   Pour in a chilled glass. Garnish with banana slices, if desired.

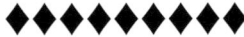

3.   Serve and enjoy!

♦♦♦♦♦♦♦♦♦

Banana Avocado and Fennel Shake

This nutrition-packed smoothie recipe with banana, avocado and fennel is a healthy and filling drink that will give you the energy and immunity boost you need.

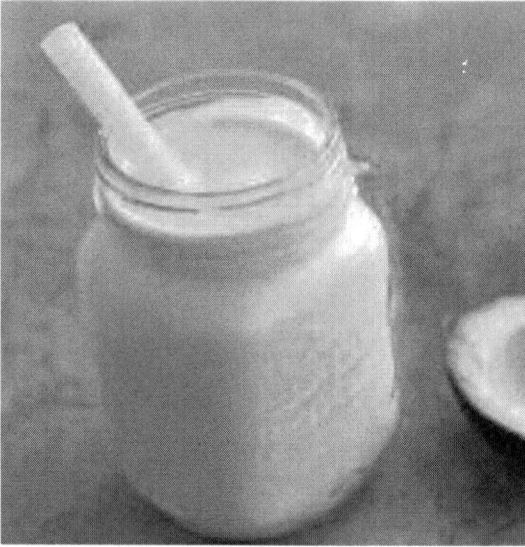

Preparation Time: 5 minutes
Total Time: 5 minutes
Yield: 1 serving

Ingredients

1 small banana, cut into small pieces
¼ medium avocado, cubed
¼ medium fennel bulb, shredded

1 teaspoon honey (optional)
water to max line

Method

1.   Combine banana, watercress, avocado, honey, and water in the tall glass. Process in theNutriBullet for 20 seconds or until it becomes smooth.

2.   Pour in a serving glass. Garnish with a slice of banana or avocado, if desired.

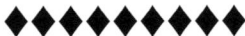

3.   Serve and enjoy!

◆◆◆◆◆◆◆◆◆

Spiced Pumpkin Almond Smoothie

This rich and delicious smoothie is just what you need to set your energy back on track during a tiresome afternoon.

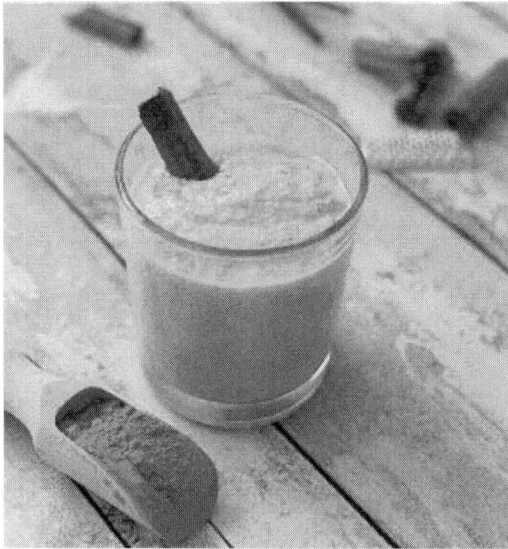

Preparation Time: 5 minutes
Total Time: 5 minutes
Yield: 1 serving

Ingredients

½ cup pumpkin puree
1 tablespoon rolled oats
1 teaspoon honey
2/3 cup almond milk

¼ teaspoon cinnamon powder
water to max line

Method

1.   Combine pumpkin, rolled oats, honey, almond milk and cinnamon in the tall glass. Process in the NutriBullet for 10-15 seconds or until mixture becomes smooth.

2.   Transfer mixture in a serving glass.

3.   Serve and enjoy!

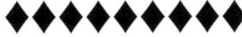

Chia Power Chocolate Strawberry Smoothie

Chia seeds are considered little miracles of the nature and they are proved to have beneficial effect on the cardiovascular system. Their taste is very mild so they won't influence the taste of the final drink.

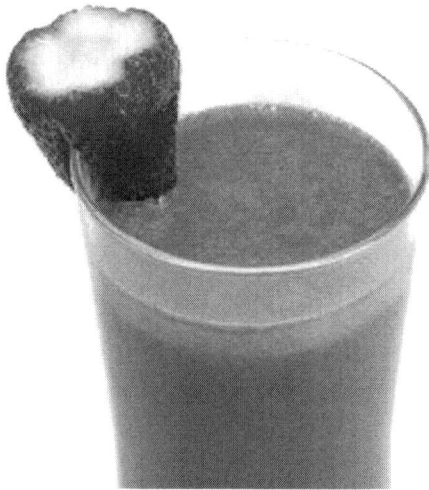

Preparation Time: 5 minutes
Total Time: 5 minutes
Yield: 1 serving

Ingredients

1 tablespoon raw cocoa powder
1 teaspoon cocoa nibs
3 pieces strawberries, halved

½ medium frozen banana
1 tablespoon chia seeds
1 teaspoon maple syrup
¾ cup almond milk

Method

1.   Combine all ingredients in the tall glass. Process in the NutriBullet for 20 seconds or until mixture becomes smooth.
2.   Transfer mixture in a serving glass.
3.   Serve and enjoy!

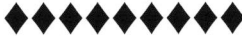

◆◆◆◆◆◆◆◆

Banana Choco Chia Smoothie

Rich and with a thick consistency, this smoothie is great to boost your energy in the morning. Plus, having such a high fiber content, it will keep you full for a longer period of time.

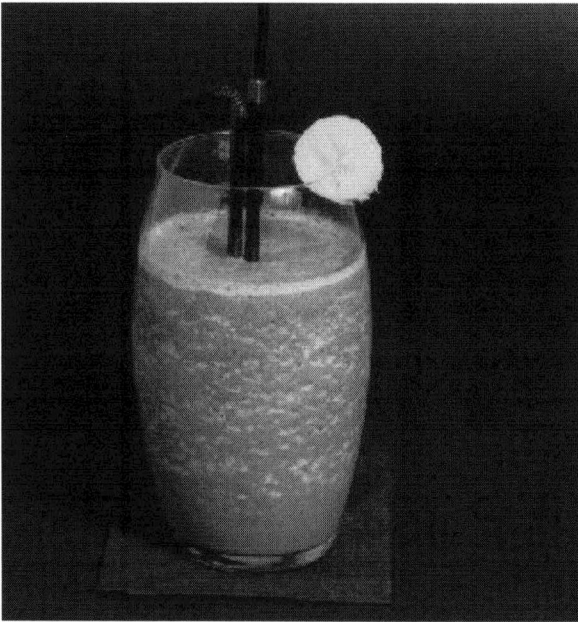

Preparation Time: 5 minutes
Total Time: 5 minutes
Yield:1 serving

Ingredients
1 mediumfrozen banana, peeled and cut

1 tablespoon raw cocoa powder
½ cup almond milk
¼ cup yogurt, vanilla flavored
1 tablespoon chia seeds

Method

1.   Combine banana, cocoa, milk, yogurt and chia seeds in the tall glass. Process in the NutriBullet for 20 seconds or until mixture becomes smooth.
2.   Transfer mixture in a serving glass.
3.   Serve and enjoy!

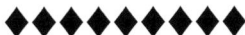

◆◆◆◆◆◆◆◆◆

Cucumber Honeydew and Yogurt Smoothie

This smoothie recipe with cucumber, honeydew melon, lime, and yogurt makes a nutritious and filling snack best when the weather is hot.

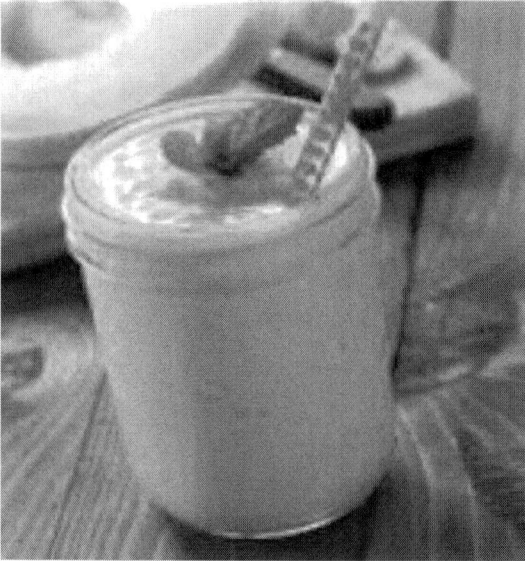

Preparation Time: 5 minutes
Total Time: 5 minutes
Yield: 1 serving

Ingredients

1 cup honeydew melon, cubed
½ medium cucumber, deseeded, diced
½ cup Greek yogurt, plain or vanilla

1 tablespoon lemon juice
1 teaspoon agave nectar (optional)
water to max line

Method

1.	Place honeydew, cucumber, Greek yogurt, lemon juice, agave nectar, and water into the tall glass. Process in the NutriBullet for 20 seconds or until becomes smooth.
2.	Pour in a chilled serving glass. Garnish with mint sprig or a slice of cucumber, if desired.
3.	Serve and enjoy!

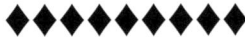

◆◆◆◆◆◆◆◆◆

Raspberry Cucumber and Lemon Blast

Thishealthy smoothiewith raspberries, cucumber, and lemon is so refreshing and delicious.

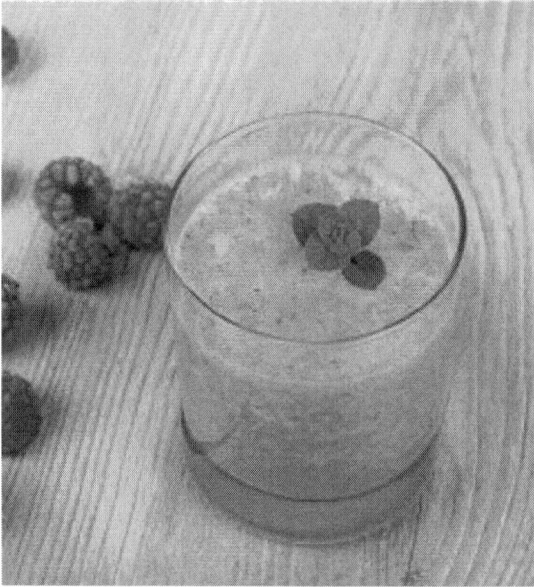

Preparation Time: 5 minutes
Total Time: 5 minutes
Yield:1 serving

Ingredients

¾ cup frozen raspberries
¼ medium cucumber, sliced

1 tablespoon lemon juice
½ cup Greek yogurt
1 teaspoon honey
water to max line

Method

1.   Combineraspberries, cucumber, lemon juice, yogurt, honey, and water in the tall glass. Process in the NutriBullet for 20 seconds or until becomes smooth.

2.   Pour in a chilled serving glass. Garnish with mint sprig, if desired.

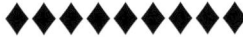

3.   Serve and enjoy!

♦♦♦♦♦♦♦♦♦

Cucumber Wheatgrass and Banana Smoothie

If you are looking for a beverage that has all the nutrients you need to keep your body organs healthy this is the recipe for you. This juice is made with pineapple wheatgrass, coconut water and honey.

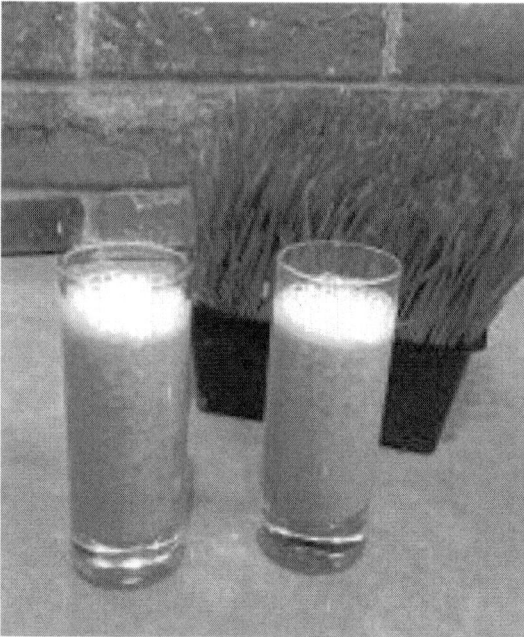

Preparation Time: 5 minutes
Total Time: 5 minutes
Yield:1 serving

Ingredients

1 handful of wheat grass
½ medium cucumber, cut into small pieces
1 medium banana, sliced
1 teaspoon honey
coconutwater to max line

Method

1.   Place wheatgrass, cucumber, banana, honey, and coconut water in the tall glass. Process in the NutriBullet for 10-12 seconds or until combined well.

2.   Pour in a serving glass. Garnish with banana or cucumber slices, if desired.

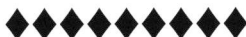

3.   Serve and enjoy!

◆◆◆◆◆◆◆◆◆

Grapefruit Yogurt and Chia Smoothie

Grapefruit is so refreshing, delicious and nutritious! But they really shine combined with a touch of mint and some vanilla yogurt.

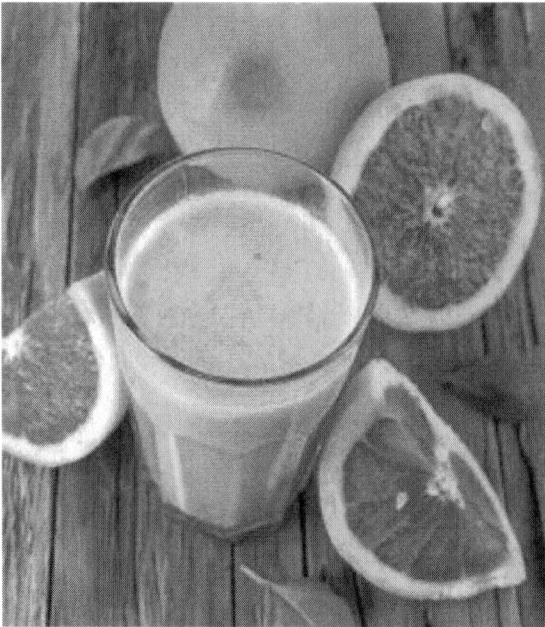

Preparation Time: 5 minutes
Total Time: 5 minutes
Yield: 1 serving

Ingredients
1 medium grapefruit, cut into segments
½ cup vanilla yogurt
½ tablespoon chia seeds
2 ice cubes
1 teaspoon maple syrup (optional)
water to max line

Method
1.   Combine grapefruit, yogurt, chia seeds, ice cubes, maple syrup and water in the tall glass. Process in the NutriBullet for 20-30 seconds or until mixture becomes smooth.
2.   Pour mixture in a serving glass.
3.   Serve and enjoy!

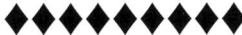

Blueberry Apple and Coconut Blast

This awesome smoothie recipe is good for the heart because it is rich in fiber and antioxidants.

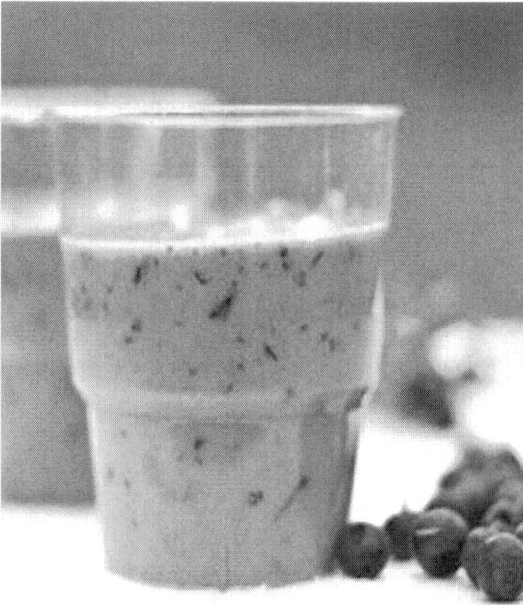

Preparation Time: 5 minutes
Total Time: 5 minutes
Yield:1 serving

Ingredients
½ cup fresh blueberries
1 medium apple, cored and diced
2 tablespoon coconut milk
2 ice cubes
coconut water to max line

Method
1.   Combine blueberries, apple, coconut milk, ice cubes, and coconut water in the tall glass. Process in the NutriBullet for 20-30 seconds or until mixture becomes smooth.
2.   Transfer mixture in a serving glass.
3.   Serve and enjoy!

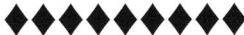

◆◆◆◆◆◆◆◆

Green Kiwi Smoothie

Green smoothies are loaded with nutrients and this particular drink makes no exception. Spinach and kale come together with lime and kiwi to create a drink that can be served at any time of the day for an energy and nutritional boost.

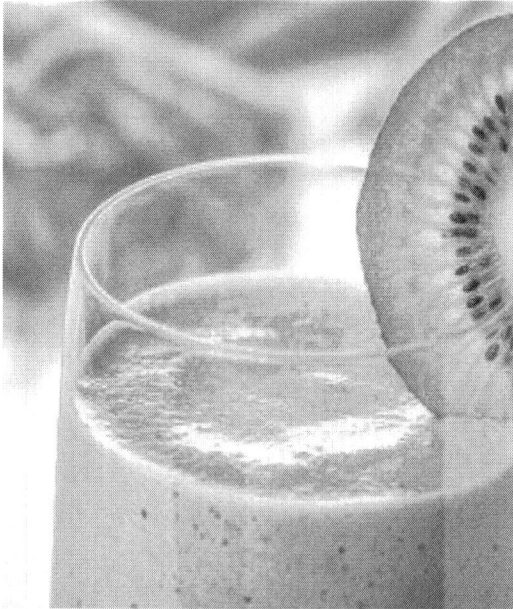

Preparation Time: 5 minutes
Total Time: 5 minutes
Yield: 1 serving

Ingredients
1 medium kiwi fruit, peeled
1 cup fresh baby spinach
1 cup kale, shredded
1 teaspoon agave syrup
2 tablespoonslime juice
coconut water to max line

Method
1.   Combine kiwi, spinach, kale, agave syrup, lime juice, and coconut water in the tall glass. Process in the NutriBullet for 10-15 seconds or until mixture becomes smooth.
2.   Pour mixture in a serving glass.
3.   Serve and enjoy!

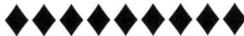

◆◆◆◆◆◆◆◆◆

Apple Celery Cucumber and Green Tea Blast

Green tea is one of the healthiest teas out there. It is refreshing and packed with vitamins and antioxidants. One glass of green tea every day will improve your health.

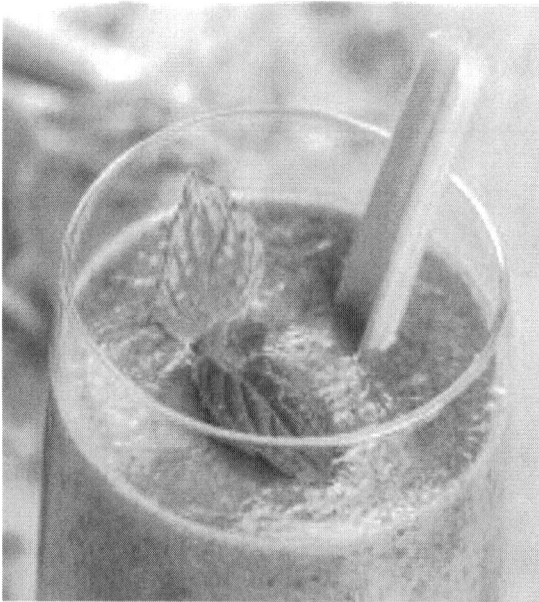

Preparation Time: 5 minutes
Total Time: 5 minutes
Yield: 1 serving

Ingredients
1 medium apple, cored and diced
2 celery stalks, diced
½ medium cucumber, sliced
freshly brewed green tea to max line

Method
1.   Combine apple, celery, cucumber, and green tea in the tall glass. Process in the NutriBullet for 20 seconds or until mixture becomes smooth.
2.   Transfer mixture in a serving glass.
3.   Serve and enjoy!

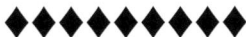

◆◆◆◆◆◆◆◆

Cereal Berry and Banana Blast

This delicious and nutritious smoothie recipe can help regulate blood pressure prevent cardiovascular disease.

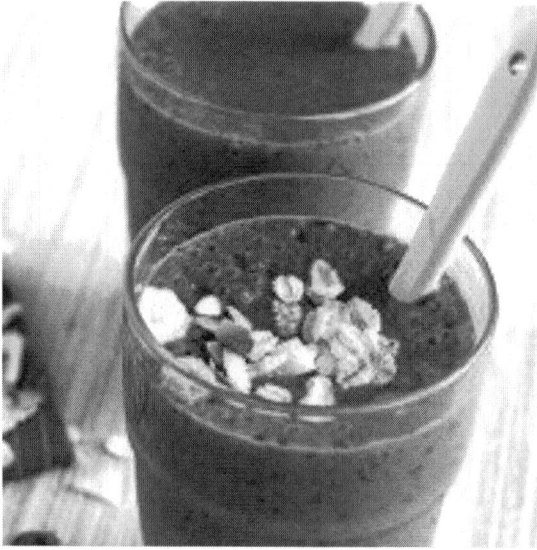

Preparation Time: 5 minutes
Total Time: 5 minutes
Yield:1 serving

Ingredients
3 tablespoonsgranola

2/3 cup mixed berries
½ cup plain yogurt
¼ cup crushed ice
1 teaspoon honey

Method

1.   Combine granola, mixed berries, yogurt, ice and honey in the tall glass. Process in the NutriBullet for 20 seconds or until mixture becomes smooth.
2.   Pour mixture in a serving glass.
3.   Serve and enjoy!

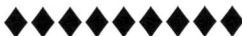

◆◆◆◆◆◆◆◆◆

Blueberry Yogurt Smoothie Recipe

Yogurt smoothie recipes are very versatile. You can simplyadd any kind of fruits and/or vegetables you want and make a delicious, healthy andfilling smoothie to enjoy anytime of the day. The fiber in theblueberries and the protein in yogurt makes a perfect combination for optimum health.

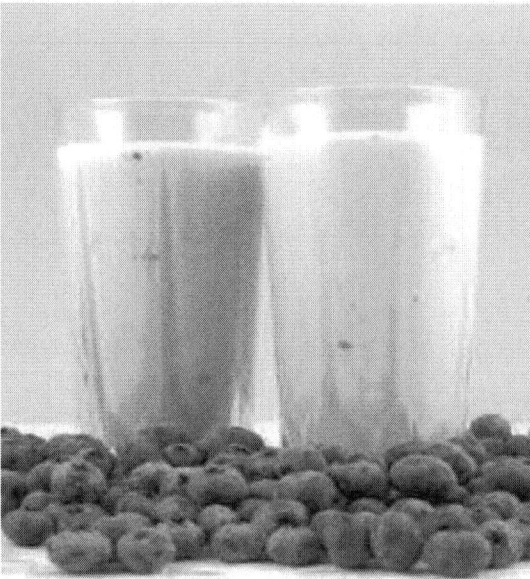

Preparation Time: 5 minutes
Total Time: 5 minutes

Yield:1 serving

Ingredients
½ cup blueberries
½ cup Greek yogurt
½ cup organic milk
1 teaspoon honey

Method
1.   Place blueberries, yogurt, organic milk, and honey in your Nutribullet and process 15-20 seconds until smooth and creamy.
2.   Pour in a glass and serve immediately

Tip:

•   Replace the blueberries with raspberries or strawberries and create a new drink.

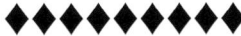

♦♦♦♦♦♦♦♦♦

Blueberry Kombucha Smoothie

Blueberries have good nutritional profile and contains high amount of antioxidants. Their flavor works great with the Kombucha and the final drink taste better than any store bought drink you might think of.

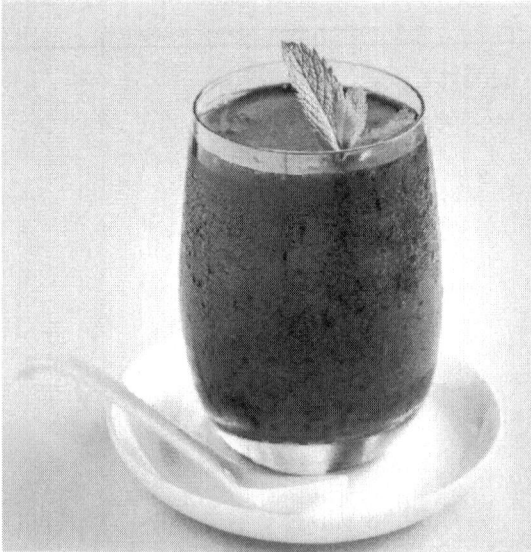

Preparation Time: 5 minutes
Total Time: 5 minutes
Yield:1 serving

Ingredients
½ cup frozen blueberries
1 medium banana, cut into small pieces
1 teaspoon honey
Kombucha tea to max line

Method
1.   Place blueberries, banana, honey, Kombucha in the Nutribullet.
2.   Process for 10-15 seconds or until smooth.
3.   Transfer mixture in a serving glass. Enjoy.

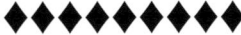

◆◆◆◆◆◆◆◆◆

Tropical Duo Blast

Everyone loves tropical fruits and this recipe gives you the taste of two fruits combined into a drink that is delicious and nutritious.

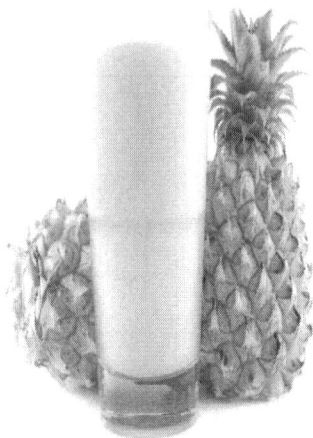

Preparation Time: 5 minutes
Total Time: 5 minutes
Yield: 1 serving

Ingredients

½ cup mango, cubed
½ cup pineapple juice
1 tablespoon wheat germ
2 tablespoons coconut milk
coconutwater to max line

Method

1.   Combine all the ingredients in your Nutribullet and process for 20-30 seconds or until well blended and smooth.
2.   Pour in a glass of your choice and serve right away.

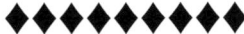

♦♦♦♦♦♦♦♦♦

Blackberry Banana Oatmeal Smoothie

The nice flavor and nutrition of the blueberries,banana, and oatmeal make this smoothie perfect for breakfast or snack. Being so rich in healthy carbs and other important nutrients, it will give you an instant energy boost and will also keep you feeling satisfied for a longer period of time.

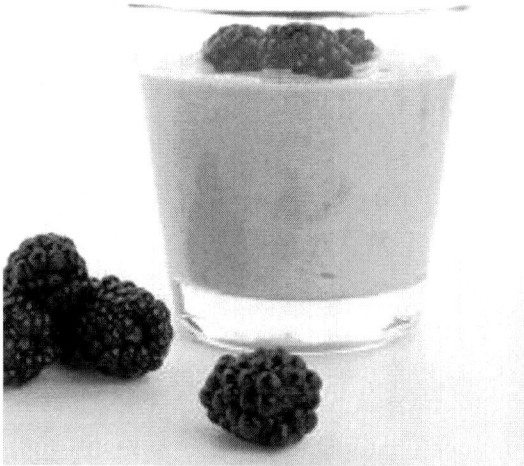

Preparation Time: 5 minutes
Total Time: 5 minutes

Yield:1 serving

Ingredients
½ cup blackberries
½ medium banana, cut into small pieces
¼ cup oatmeal, cooked
½ cup organic milk
1 teaspoon honey

Method
1.   Combine blackberries, banana, oatmeal, milk, and honey in your Nutribullet and process until well blended and smooth.
2.   Pour in a glass of your choice and enjoy.

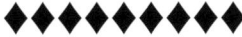

◆◆◆◆◆◆◆◆◆

Strawberry Almond and Kiwi Blast with Chia

Berries and kiwi fruits have are naturally rich in vitamin C and other antioxidants so imagine how good this smoothie is!

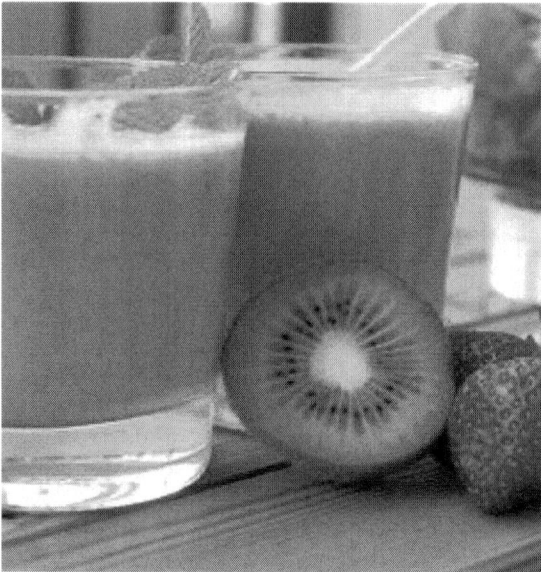

Preparation Time: 5 minutes
Total Time: 5 minutes
Yield:1 serving

Ingredients

½ cup strawberries, sliced
1 medium kiwi fruit, peeled, sliced
½ cup vanilla yogurt
½ cup almond milk
1 teaspoon honey
1 teaspoon chia seeds

Method

1.   Combine all the ingredients in your Nutribullet and process until the drink is well blended and smooth.
2.   Pour it in a glass of your choice and drink right away.

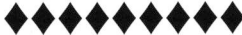

◆◆◆◆◆◆◆◆

Pineapple Banana and Mango Blast

Fresh and delicious, this smoothie will awaken your taste buds. It's loaded with antioxidants and vitamins, a great way to start your day or brighten up your afternoon.

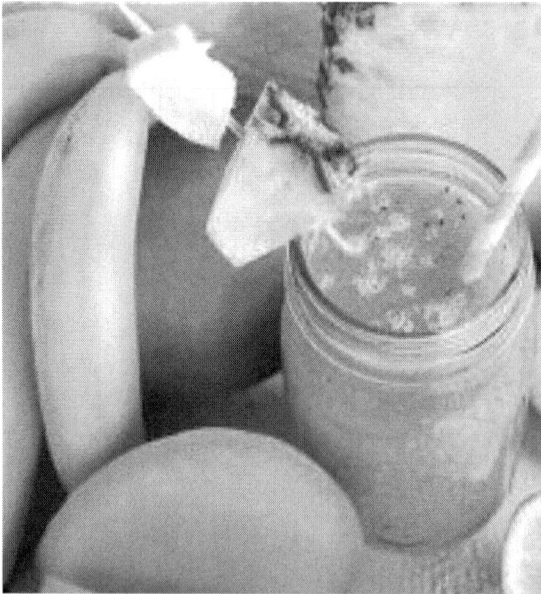

Preparation Time: 5 minutes
Total Time: 5 minutes
Yield:1 serving

Ingredients
½ cup pineapple chunks
½ medium frozen banana, cut into small pieces
½ cup ripe mango diced
2/3 cup almond milk

Method
1.   Place the pineapple, banana, mango, and almond milk in the Nutribullet.
2.   Process for 20 seconds or until smooth.
3.   Pour mixture in a serving glass. Enjoy.

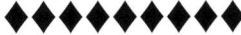

◆◆◆◆◆◆◆◆◆

Yummy Dragonfruit Yogurt and Almond Smoothie

The almondmilk combines perfectly with the dragonfruit, creating a delicious smoothie.Great to share with the entire family.

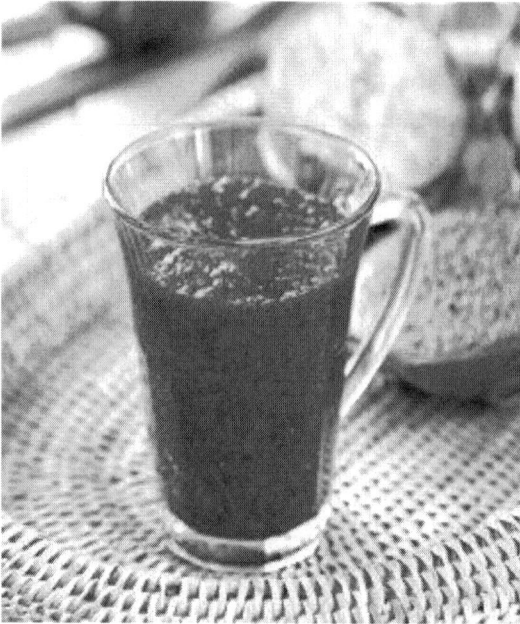

Preparation Time: 5 minutes
Total Time: 5 minutes
Yield:1 serving

Ingredients

1 medium dragonfruit, peeled and cut
into small pieces
½ cup vanilla yogurt
½ almond milk
dash of cinnamon

Method

1.   Place the dragonfruit, yogurt,
almond milk, and cinnamon in the
Nutribullet.
2.   Process for 10-15 seconds or until
smooth.
3.   Transfer in a serving glass. Enjoy.

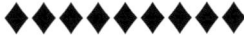

◆◆◆◆◆◆◆◆◆

Easy Papaya Fennel and Pineapple Blast

This smoothie recipe combines the flavor and nutrition of papaya, pineapple and fennel. It makes a wonderful refreshment that is also heart friendly.

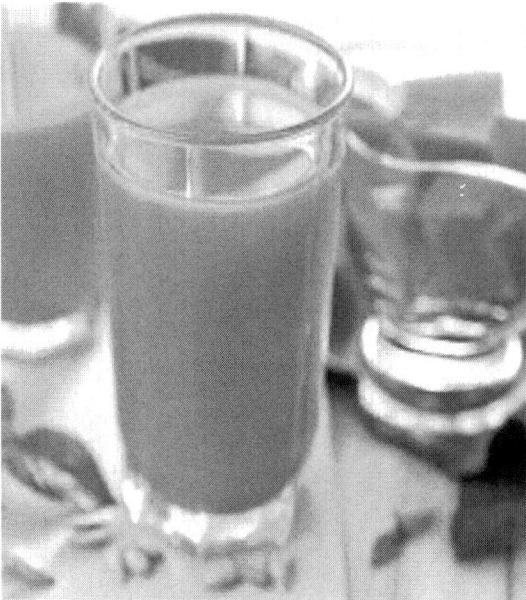

Preparation Time: 5 minutes
Total Time: 5 minutes
Yield:1 serving

Ingredients
2/3 cup papaya, cubed
¼ medium fennel bulb, shredded
½ cup pineapple juice
1 teaspoon agave nectar
coconut water to max line

Method
1.   Place papaya, fennel, pineapple,
agave nectar, and water in the Nutribullet.
2.   Process for 20 seconds or until
smooth.
3.   Pour in a serving glass. Enjoy.

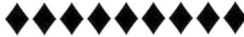

◆◆◆◆◆◆◆◆

Berry Pecan and Maple Smoothie

Another truly irresistible fruity smoothie with berries, pecans, and maple syrup.

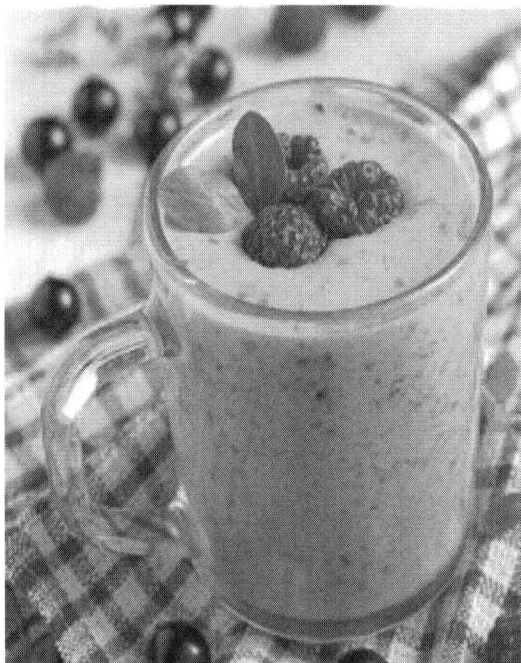

Preparation Time: 5 minutes
Total Time: 5 minutes
Yield: 1 serving

Ingredients

½ cup frozen mixed berries
6 pecans
1 tablespoon lime juice
1 teaspoon maple syrup
almond milk to max line

Method

1.   Place berries, pecans, lime juice, maple syrup, and almond milk in the Nutribullet.
2.   Process for 20 seconds or until smooth.
3.   Transfer in a serving glass. Enjoy.

Tip

You can also use soy milk or organic milk as a substitute for almond milk.

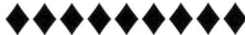

◆◆◆◆◆◆◆◆◆

Beet Blueberry and Coconut Smoothie

Beets are rich in antioxidants and when combined with blackberries they yield a delicious and nutritious smoothie that also has a beautiful color.

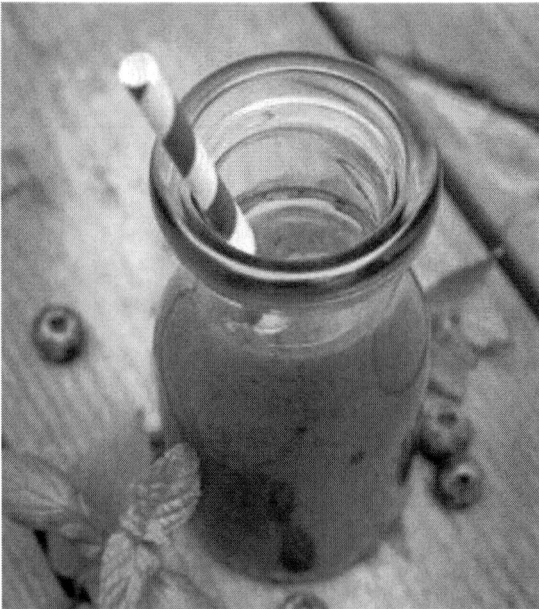

Preparation Time: 5 minutes
Total Time: 5 minutes
Yield: 1 servings

Ingredients
1 piece beetroot, diced
½ cup blueberries
2 tablespoon coconut milk
1 teaspoon honey
coconut water to max line

Method
1.   Place beetroot, blueberries, honey, and coconut water in the Nutribullet.
2.   Process for 20 seconds or until smooth.
3.   Transfer in a serving glass. Enjoy.

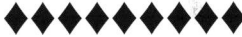

◆◆◆◆◆◆◆◆

Plum Banana and Almond Smoothie

This smoothie is all about the flavor plum, banana, and almond. It is delicious and rich in fiber content.

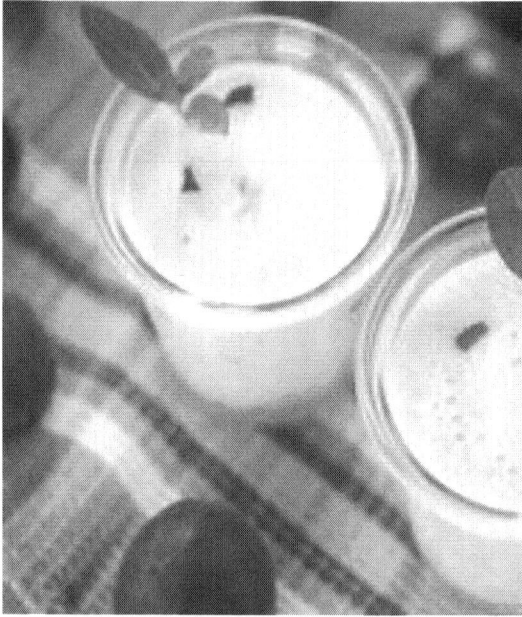

Preparation Time: 5 minutes
Total Time: 5 minutes
Yield: 1 serving

Ingredients
2 pieces plum, diced
½ medium frozen banana, sliced
½ cup almond milk
1 teaspoon flaxseeds

Method
1.   Place the plum, banana, almond milk, and flaxseeds in the Nutribullet.
2.   Process for 20 seconds or until smooth.
3.   Pour in a serving glass. Enjoy.

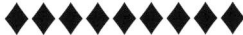

◆◆◆◆◆◆◆◆

Spiced Banana Walnut Smoothie

This smoothie has banana and cinnamon flavor and combined with walnuts, this smoothie yield a drink that tastes great and has enough nutrients to give you an energy boost when you are running low.

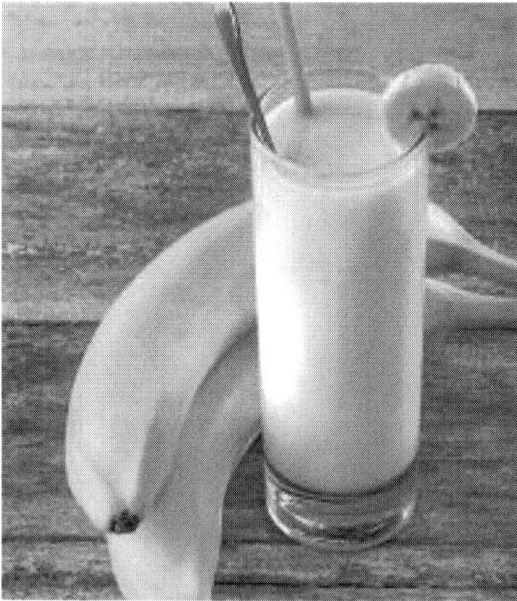

Preparation Time: 5 minutes
Total Time: 5 minutes
Yield: 1 serving

Ingredients
1 medium banana, cut into small pieces
6 pieces walnuts, coarsely chopped
½ cup yogurt
½ cup skim milk
2 ice cubes
dash of ground cinnamon

Method
1.   Place banana, walnuts, yogurt, skim milk, ice cubes, and cinnamon in the Nutribullet.
2.   Process for 20-30 seconds or until smooth.
3.   Transfer in a serving glass. Enjoy.

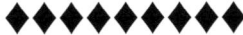

◆◆◆◆◆◆◆◆◆

Banana Walnut and Kale Smoothie

This green smoothie recipe with banana, walnuts, and kale is a must have especially when you want to have a healthy heart because it is rich in fiber and potassium.

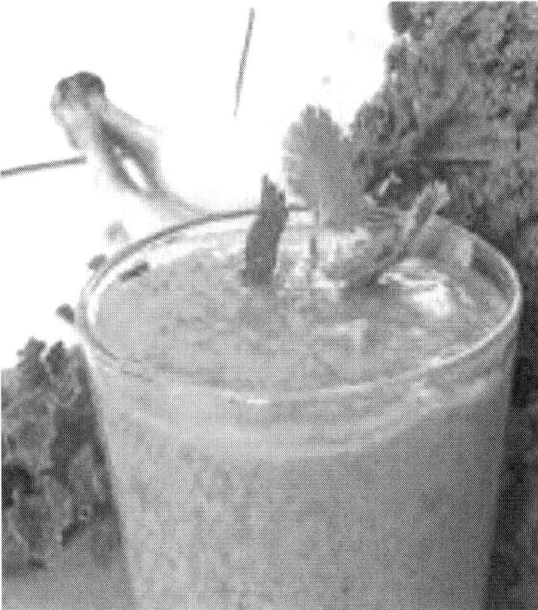

Preparation Time: 5 minutes
Total Time: 5 minutes
Yield:1 serving

Ingredients

1 medium banana, cut into small pieces
1cup kale, torn
2 tablespoons walnuts, chopped
coconutwater to max line
dash of nutmeg, to serve

Method

1.   Combine banana, kale, walnuts, coconut water, and nutmeg in the tall glass. Process in the NutriBullet for 10-15 seconds or until it becomes smooth.
2.   Pour in a serving glass. Garnish with a small slice of banana. Sprinkle with nutmeg.
3.   Serve and enjoy!

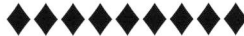

◆◆◆◆◆◆◆◆◆

Banana Turmeric Yogurt Smoothie Recipe

This smoothie recipe with banana and turmeric has many health benefits to the body.

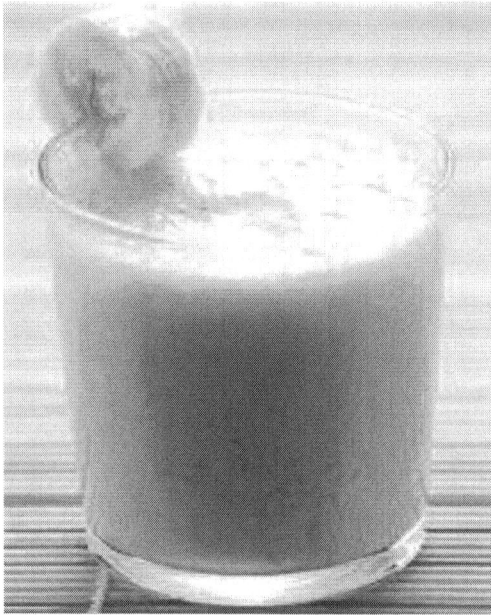

Preparation Time: 5 minutes
Total Time: 5 minutes
Yield:1 serving

Ingredients
1 medium banana, cut into small pieces
½ cup Greek yogurt
½ cup organic milk
1 tablespoon lemon juice
pinchof turmeric powder

Method
1.   Place banana, yogurt, milk, lemon juice, and turmeric in the Nutribullet.
2.   Process for 10-15 seconds or until smooth.
3.   Transfer in a serving glass. Enjoy.

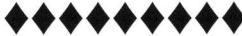

◆◆◆◆◆◆◆◆

Peanut Butter Banana Kale Smoothie with Cinnamon

This green smoothie recipe with banana, peanut butter, kale and cinnamon is a must have especially when you are feeling under the weather; it will supply you with essential nutrients to help you recover from illness.

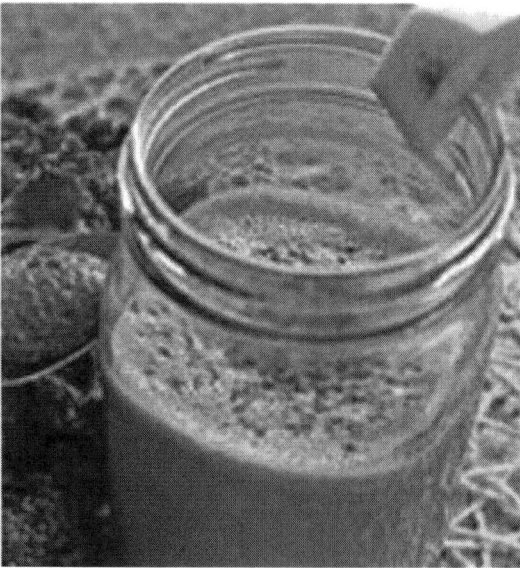

Preparation Time: 5 minutes
Total Time: 5 minutes
Yield: 1 serving

Ingredients

2 tablespoons peanut butter
1 medium banana, cut into small pieces
1cup kale, torn
water to max line
dash of ground cardamom, to serve

Method

1.   Combine peanut butter, banana, kale, water, and cardamom in the tall glass. Process in the NutriBullet for 10-15 seconds or until it becomes smooth.
2.   Pour in a serving glass. Garnish with a small slice of banana and sprinkle with cinnamon.
3.   Serve and enjoy!

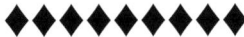

♦♦♦♦♦♦♦♦♦

Easy Avocado Citrus Smoothie

This wonderful green smoothie made with avocado, banana, grapefruit, and honey is so delicious that you will keep on having it for a power-packed breakfast or grab and go snack.

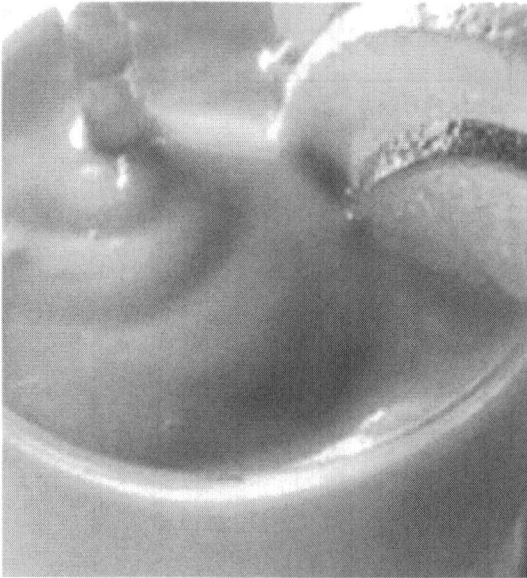

Preparation Time: 5 minutes
Total Time: 5 minutes
Yield:1 serving

Ingredients
¼ medium ripe avocado, diced
1 medium orange, cut into segments
1 tablespoon lime juice
1 teaspoon honey
almond milk to max line

Method
1.   Combine the avocado, orange segments, lime juice, honey, and almond milk in the tall glass. Process in the NutriBullet for 10-15 seconds or until becomes smooth and creamy.
2.   Pour mixture in a serving glass. Garnish with a slice of orange and lime, if desired.
3.   Serve and enjoy!

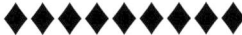

◆◆◆◆◆◆◆◆◆

Goji Berry Peach Raspberry and Yogurt Smoothie

This delectable yogurt smoothie recipe made with Goji berries, peach and yogurt is packed with all the good for you nutrients to keep you healthy and strong.

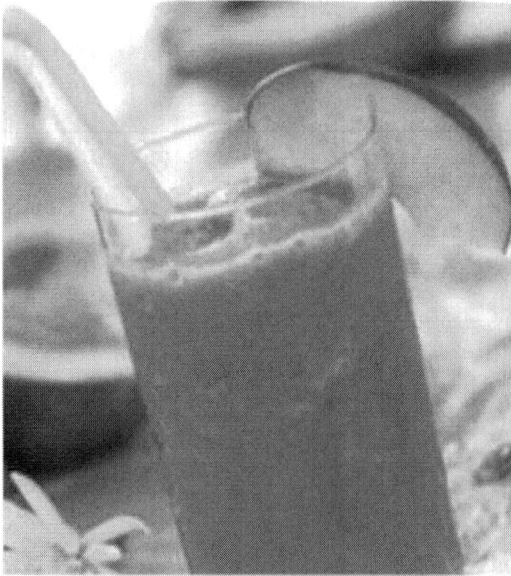

Preparation Time: 5 minutes
Total Time: 5 minutes
Yield:1 serving

Ingredients
1 medium peach, diced
½ cup raspberries
2 tablespoons Goji Berries
½ cup Greek yogurt, plain
water to max line

Method
1.　　Combine the peach, raspberries, Goji berries, yogurt, and water in the tall glass. Process in the NutriBullet for 20 seconds or until it becomes smooth.
2.　　Pour mixture in a serving glass. Garnish with a slice of peach, if desired.
3.　　Serve and enjoy!

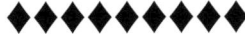

◆◆◆◆◆◆◆◆

Flaxseeds Oat and Fig Smoothie

Flaxseeds are miracle seeds because they contain good amounts of healthy fats and fiber and when combined with oats and figs it makes a filling and delicious drink.

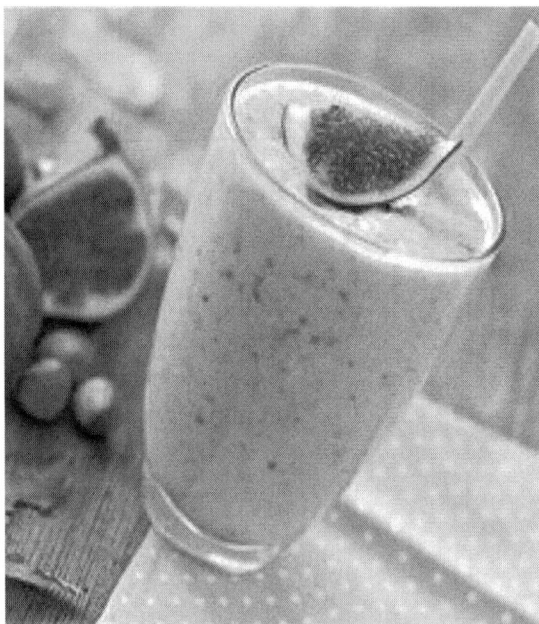

Preparation Time: 5 minutes
Total Time: 5 minutes
Yield:1 serving

Ingredients

½ cup oatmeal, cooked
1 medium fig, cut into small pieces
2 teaspoons flaxseeds
1 teaspoon honey
½ cup almond milk

Method

1.   Place oatmeal, fig, flaxseeds, honey, and almond milk in your Nutribullet and process 20 seconds or until smooth.
2.   Pour in a glass of your choice and drink right away.

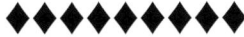

◆◆◆◆◆◆◆◆

Easy Apricot Yogurt and Vanilla Smoothie

The smoothie is thick and highly nourishing, perfect to start a day on a high note or simply have a healthy afternoon snack.

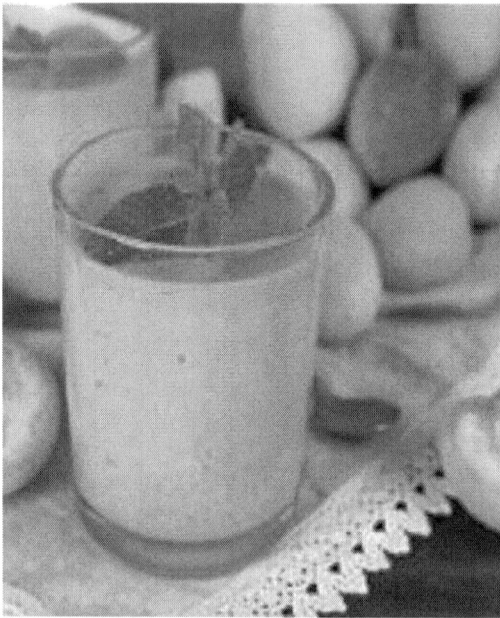

Preparation Time: 5 minutes
Total Time: 5 minutes
Yield:1 serving

Ingredients
3 pieces apricots, cut into small pieces
½ cup Greek yogurt
½ cup almond milk
¼ teaspoon vanilla extract
1-2 ice cubes

Method
1.   Combine apricots, yogurt, almond milk, vanilla extract, and ice cubes in your Nutribullet. Process until well combined and smooth.
2.   Pour in a glass of your choice and serve immediately.

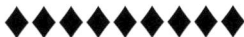

◆◆◆◆◆◆◆◆◆

Dates Raspberry and Almond Smoothie

This smoothie with dates, raspberries, and almond milk is packed with antioxidants and fiber which can lower blood cholesterol levels.

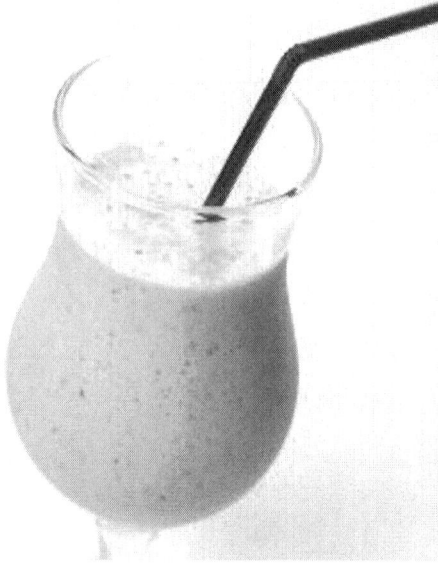

Preparation Time: 5 minutes
Total Time: 5 minutes
Yield: 1 serving

Ingredients
3 pieces dates, pitted
½ cup frozen raspberries
½ cup almond milk
2 tablespoons wheat germ

Method
1.   Combine dates, raspberries, almond milk, and wheat germ in your Nutribullet. Process until well blended and smooth.
2.   Pour in a glass of your choice and serve.

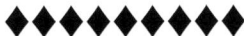

◆◆◆◆◆◆◆◆◆

Mango Orange Pineapple Smoothie

This fiber-rich smoothie recipe with mango, orange and pineapple will give you a taste of the tropics and energy boost!

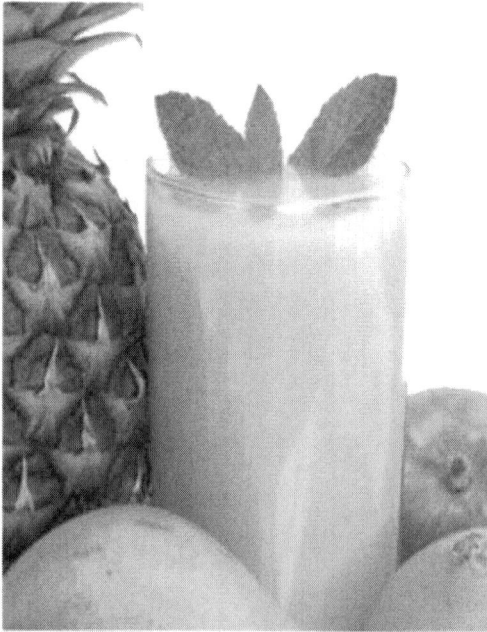

Preparation Time: 5 minutes
Total Time: 5 minutes
Yield: 1 serving

Ingredients
½ cup mango, cubed
½ cup pineapple, cubed
½ medium orange, cut into segments
1-2 ice cubes
½ cup coconut water to max line

Method
1.   Place mango, pineapple, orange, ice, and coconut water into the tall glass. Process in the NutriBullet for 20-30 seconds or until combined well.
2.   Pour in a chilled glass. Garnish with a small chunk of pineapple or a slice of orange, if desired.
3.   Serve and enjoy!

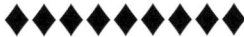

♦♦♦♦♦♦♦♦♦

Mango Carrot Ginger and Lime Juice

This healthy drink with mango, carrot, and lime will help give you the energy and nutrients you need to meet your daily requirements.

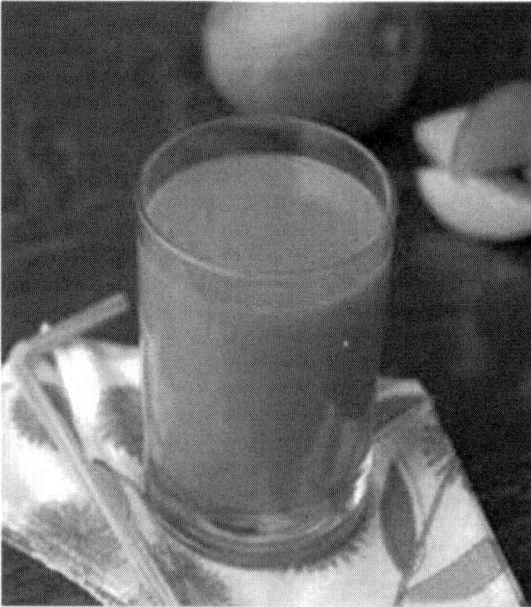

Preparation Time: 5 minutes
Total Time: 5 minutes
Yield: 1 serving

Ingredients

1 medium carrot, cut into small pieces
½ cup mango, cubed
1 tablespoon lime juice
½ teaspoon ginger, grated
water to max line

Method

1.   Combine carrot, mango, lime juice, and ginger in the tall glass. Process in the NutriBullet for 20-30 seconds or until smooth.
2.   Pour in a serving glass. Garnish with a slice of mango, if desired.
3.   Serve and enjoy!

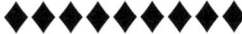

♦♦♦♦♦♦♦♦

Mango Banana and Almond Smoothie

This smoothie recipe with mango, banana, wheat germ, and almond milk is so delicious that you will want to make some more. It is also packed with important nutrients that can promote heart health.

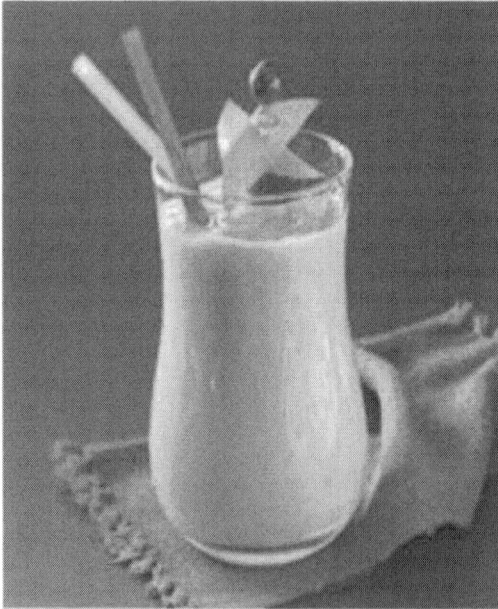

Preparation Time: 5 minutes
Total Time: 5 minutes
Yield: 1 serving

Ingredients
½ medium mango, cubed
½ medium banana, cut into small pieces
1 tablespoon wheat germ
3/4 cup almond milk

Method
1.   Combine mango, banana, wheat germ, and almond milk in the tall glass. Process in the NutriBullet for 20 seconds or until it becomes smooth.
2.   Pour in a serving glass. Garnish with a small slice of mango, if desired.
3.   Serve and enjoy!

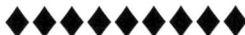

◆◆◆◆◆◆◆◆

Banana Lemon and Yogurt Smoothie

This another refreshing quick and easy blasts for losing weight perfect accompaniment for hot day.

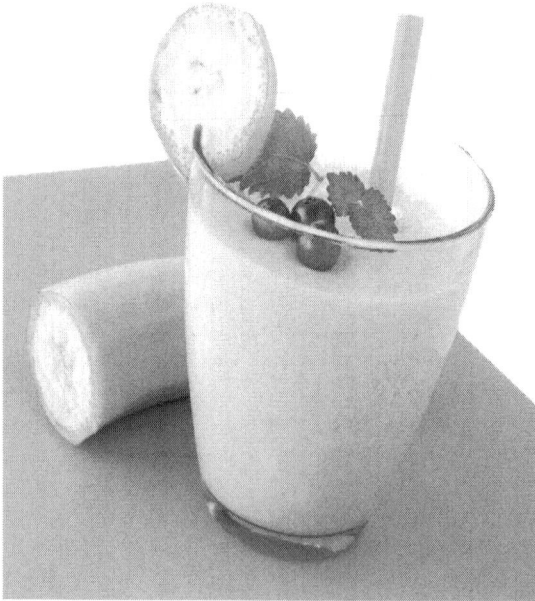

Preparation Time: 5 minutes
Total Time: 5 minutes
Yield:1 serving

Ingredients

½ cup lemonade
1 medium banana, cut into small pieces
½ cup Greek yogurt
1-2 ice cubes

Method

1.   Combine the lemonade, banana, yogurt, and ice cubes in the Nutribullet.
2.   Process for 20-30 seconds or until smooth.
3.   Transfer in a serving glass.
4.   Enjoy.

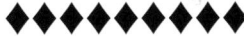

◆◆◆◆◆◆◆◆

Printed in Great Britain
by Amazon.co.uk, Ltd.,
Marston Gate.

14591054R00117